Contents

About the author

Dr Barry Jones was the first consultant paediatrician at Moorfields Eye Hospital London, and the consultant in charge of the Donald Winnicott Centre at Queen Elizabeth Hospital for Children in Hackney, a centre for the assessment and managment of disabled children.

In 1991 he was awarded the Jeanette Lappe Memorial Prize in Bio-Ethics by the Hastings Center, New York, and he subsequently received the Sense Award 2001 for exceptional achievement in the field of deaf blindness.

He is now retired from full-time practice, but continues to participate in projects involving visually impaired children in Southern India.

Acknowledgements

This book is based on a PhD thesis submitted to the University of Wales, and I would first of all wish to thank my supervisor, Dr Hugh Upton, for the considerable help that he gave me in writing it, and for his unfailing patience during its elephantine gestation. I would particularly like to thank Dr Harry Lesser, the external examiner of the thesis, who went out of his way to encourage me to publish it.

Secondly, I must thank my family for their patience over the years, in particular my wife, Dorothee, without whose support and encouragement it would not have been written at all. My daughter Katherine devoted long hours to reading and criticising the manuscript, and is responsible for eliminating most of my grammatical errors.

Most of all, I must thank my patients and their families, particularly those who belong to the ultra-orthodox Jewish community in North London, who took a great interest in the progress of 'my book' and were unstinting in their efforts to instruct me in their beliefs. I hope that they would feel that I have been fair in my comments, and would accept that this work was done with affection for them and their children.

Lastly, the staff at Radcliffe Medical Press, in particular Gillian Nineham and Jamie Etherington, have been indispensable in guiding me through the intricacies of turning a thesis into a book.

Barry Jones
May 2003

For Dorothee

Chapter 1

Introduction

This book aims to study the problems inherent in the medical, social and educational management of children with developmental disability in populations which have value systems different from that of the majority culture, using as an example a group of Hasidic Jews. Although this is a relatively small minority, the problems that they present are common to most very orthodox religious groups. The impetus for this study arose out of the practical necessity of providing for the children of such a cultural and religious group without significantly compromising the quality of the care given, unjustifiably diverting resources from other patients or, as far as possible, offending the religious susceptibilities of the group. All members of the group live in Hackney, one of the most deprived inner-city boroughs of London. All resources (medical, social and educational) are in short supply. In contrast, indicators of deprivation – unemployment, broken homes, child abuse and appalling housing – are among the highest in England. Recent figures based on the Deprivation Index[1,2] show that it is the third worst borough in England.[3] In addition, it is an area with many different ethnic and religious groups, speaking over 150 languages. One such group, accounting for about 12% of the population of the borough, are Jews, of whom about 50% are Hasidic. Among the Hasidim, marriages are arranged within small subunits of the community, and family size averages about eight children, although anything up to 15 or 20 children is not uncommon.[4]

Among the Hasidic communities, strict and total adherence to the Law of God as revealed in the Torah and other Scriptures is paramount, since only if all Jews obey all the Laws will the Messiah come. Since in at least one group, namely the Lubavitchers, there was widespread belief that their leader, the Rebbe, was waiting to declare himself to be the Messiah, such obedience has been a matter of immediate cosmic significance.[5] That he did not do so before he died reflects on the ability of the community to obey the law. Therefore any advice which tends to tempt them to disobey the Law is anathema.

As part of the adherence to Jewish law, the children (about 3200 in total) attend a variety of private Jewish schools,[4] where in most cases the emphasis is on religious education, with secular education amounting to only the minimum required by the State. There is one school (also private) outside the borough, which is acceptable from the religious point of view to most subgroups of the Hasidic community, which caters for some children with special educational needs.

The children from this community present with a wide range of developmental disabilities, including cerebral palsy and Down syndrome. Despite the small gene pool from which matings occur, there is little autosomal-recessive disease, possibly because of the taboo about marrying into the family of a disabled person.[6] A phenomenon that does occur, however, because of the large family size and the reluctance to accept any form of genetic counselling or fertility control, is that of families with several disabled members. For example, several of the families have three or four boys with fragile X syndrome, a genetically determined form of mental retardation.

Providing for the needs of disabled children within such a community is difficult both because of the private nature and inflexibility of the group's own education system, and because of the refusal of most parents in the group to allow the children's needs to be met within the Local Education Authority secular schools, or indeed even within the Jewish maintained schools run by the Local Education Authority.

The first part of this book will consider the concepts of impairment, disability and handicap in general, and the influence that culture and religious belief have on them. When considering these issues, it is necessary to attempt to define not only the formal teachings of the religion on the cause and meaning of disease or disability, but also the way in which adherents of the religion interpret this teaching in their own perceptions of themselves or others as disabled people. It is also necessary to try to differentiate between those beliefs about disability that are truly the result of adherence to a particular religion, even if they are based more on superstition than on the true teachings of that religion, and those commonly held beliefs about, for example, the causation of disability, independent of religion. However strong one's adherence to a religion may be, it can never be the only factor that influences beliefs. For example, the belief that every child should be perfect, and if it is not, someone somewhere will be able to make it perfect (what I call the *broken doll syndrome*; as all broken dolls can be mended) is widespread and independent of religious affiliation. Attributing difficulties to acceptance of disability to the effect of religious adherence may therefore be a completely false explanation. To help to clarify this dilemma, comparisons of the teachings of the world's major religions and their adherents are made.

In order to justify the claims that are made in this book, it is necessary to demonstrate that adherence to the tenets of their religion by the parents, and indeed by the children themselves, interferes with orthodox treatment of the children's conditions. Furthermore, it must be shown that this is potentially to the detriment of the child, or to the detriment of the wider community, or that it presents the physician with an insuperable ethical dilemma.

The presence of a disabled child can cause problems for a family, particularly in its relationships with others in the community, as well as practical matters such as arranging marriages for the disabled child's siblings in many religious groups, not just the Hasidim. As a result of this, the family may attempt to deny either the existence of the disabled child, or the fact that he or she is disabled. These children may not receive appropriate therapy because of the parents' attitudes, which arise from their perception of the constraints that are placed on them by their religion. On the other hand, can it be said that the interests of the disabled child are best served by receiving therapy if this results in detriment to the whole family?

Within our society, parents stand in a special relationship to their children and owe them a special duty of beneficence and non-maleficence. Within the Hasidic Jewish community, as in some other strictly religious communities, there is a duty to marry and be fruitful, and it is part of the parents' duty to arrange suitable marriages so that their children can fulfil this duty. To publicise the existence of the disabled child would be an act of maleficence towards the other children, since it would reduce their ability to find suitable partners and fulfil their obligations under the law.

On the other hand, the parents' duty of beneficence extends to all their children, including the disabled child. He has a need for medical care and supervision, and they have a duty to see that he receives it, in that he is too young to exercise autonomy and get it for himself. However, the child's doctor stands in a special relationship to the child, and only secondarily through him to his parents, and thence to his siblings. Because of this, the doctor has a greater duty of beneficence and non-maleficence to the child than to his parents or siblings. To agree to the parents' request for inadequate treatment is to collude knowingly with them in pretending that they are providing the child with appropriate management and care when in fact they are not. On the other hand, do the parents have a duty to comply with orthodox medical care? Who can rightly give consent to withhold treatment? In what circumstances can this be overruled? Is the greater good of the wider family within its cultural community of greater importance than the overall good of one member of that community? Can a doctor collude with the provision of substandard care? All of these questions will be discussed in subsequent chapters but, in my opinion, refusal to acknowledge the presence of a disabled child does pose a potential problem for the physician and the wider community, as well as for the child and their family. It could be said that it borders on that of Jehovah's Witness families who refuse life-preserving blood transfusion. In the case of the Jehovah's Witnesses, there is the belief that infusion of blood actually changes the identity of the child, and it has been said that some parents would refuse to take their child home on the grounds that it would be a different child and no longer theirs. Does this constitute child abuse and does the physician here have an actual duty to intervene?

The problem of the physician colluding with the demands of the family is further illustrated by the following example. Full investigation of a profoundly retarded child with a severe behavioural and communication disorder, including chromosome analysis, has failed to show a cause for her disability. Inevitably, the stigma of having such a child within the family reduces the likelihood of her siblings finding suitable spouses. Each time that an older sibling is being considered for a partner, I am asked to provide written evidence not that the child does not have a familial disorder, but that my investigations have failed to show that she does. The normal investigations in no way exclude a familial disorder. On the other hand, it is likely that no harm will be done, since any familial disorder, if it exists, is likely to be recessive and therefore, even within the restricted gene pool, provided that they avoid marrying cousins, unlikely to be manifested in future generations. However, although my letter does not contain an overt lie, neither is it the whole truth. Since it is said to be one of the functions of a doctor to 'do no harm', and it is unlikely that harm comes from it, can it be said that in this case the end justifies the means? On the other hand, if a solution can be found that satisfies the religious needs of the community, it is more likely to be accepted. Similarly, if the therapists are known by the community to be prepared to consider religious needs to be part of the treatment plan, that plan is more likely to be accepted.

Sometimes a problem arises because the religion itself is a major part of the aetiology of the condition. For example, a boy presented at the age of 11 years with a non-organic visual loss, which is usually associated with stress. His family belonged to one of the most ultra-orthodox sects, which meant that the boy wore long ear locks and dressed in black gabardine. He hated being conspicuous, and the unwelcome and sometimes violent attention that this drew to him in the street, but he had no way out. We were able to resolve his visual problems, but not the stress that was causing them. He subsequently developed intractable hip pain which made it difficult for him to walk and therefore difficult for him to go out. No organic cause was ever found for the hip pain. Adequate treatment here was impossible, since to give up his characteristic appearance, even though it would have reduced the stress caused by his anti-Semitic persecutors, would have removed him from the community and the family. Which is the greater harm?

It could be said of this boy that his problems were not the result of his religious beliefs and those of his family, but rather they were the result of other people's reactions to them. In the case of a second child, however, who came from a family of Exclusive Brethren, and who presented with an identical stress-related visual loss, it was the stress placed on her by the strict requirements of the religion which was the precise cause of her disability. It prevented her from socialising with school friends, visiting their homes or having them back to her own house, with the ever present threat that if she rebelled she would be excluded from contact with her own family. The parents' refusal to accept this explanation also meant that treatment was impossible. Clearly the religion was a major factor in the child's illness, but risking disruption of the family could also have caused intolerable stress. Again, what is the balance of harm?

An exaggeration of this problem arises when the dictates of the religion actually create the problem. This is well illustrated by the decree from one of the smaller Hasidic sects that no baby formula could be guaranteed to be kosher, since it was not possible to be absolutely sure that it did not contain small amounts of meat, so that if a baby could not be breastfed, it could not be fed at all. If it had been ignored, this would not just have posed a problem of treatment, but it would have resulted in criminal proceedings for neglect and culpable homicide.

I have already mentioned the 'broken doll syndrome'. Consider the case of a boy with very mild hemiplegic cerebral palsy who walks with a slight limp, but otherwise shows no adverse effects. His mother is clinically depressed, but will accept no help for this. She seeks repeated assessments in order to obtain physiotherapy (which the child does not need) in order to remove the limp (which physiotherapy cannot do). This is beginning to have an adverse effect on the child by making him very conscious of a minor defect which previously did not cause him concern. I am not sure how much of this problem is to do with the fact that he is a member of a religious community, rather than being associated with the more widespread 'broken doll syndrome'. It is my impression that, although not exclusive to them, this belief is more common in societies where marriages are arranged. For example, a Hindu mother recently said to me of her 4-year-old daughter, 'It is bad enough that she wears glasses. With dislocated lenses as well, we will never get her a husband.'

In recent years, considerable effort has been put into methods of preventing the occurrence of disability. One such method is genetic counselling. Because of their attitudes to fertility limitation, this is anathema to some groups. This not only results in families with a number of disabled children, but may also interfere with the ability of members of the family to exercise an autonomous decision in the matter. For example, within a large family, several boys are developmentally delayed because of fragile X syndrome. Each girl in the family has a 50:50 chance of carrying the abnormality and passing it on to her sons. The girls may or may not show signs of carrying the abnormal chromosome. The eldest daughter is now of marriageable age, and does show signs which make it likely – as the parents agree – that she is a carrier. I have never met her. So far as I know she has not been told, and the parents refuse to allow her to be counselled or investigated until after she is married – and presumably has given birth to an affected son. In law I suppose that this has nothing to do with me, since she is not my patient. However, what is my responsibility to her and to her prospective husband? Emson[7] discusses this in relation to the similar problem of maintaining confidentiality in the case of a patient diagnosed with Huntington's disease. This is a degenerative neurological disease, the symptoms of which are not manifested until mid-adulthood, but which results in complete mental and physical breakdown and eventual death. It is inherited as an autosomal dominant, which means that the patient's children have a 50:50 chance of carrying the gene and thus manifesting the disease. He believes that, as I have suggested above, to deny this information to the children of the patient interferes with their ability to exercise autonomy. He therefore argues that the patient has a duty to restrict his own autonomy in the interest of that of his children, and furthermore, that if he does not accept this duty, this imposes a duty on his physician to break confidentiality. The latter duty is restricted to disclosing only that which is necessary for the children to exercise autonomy. If this is applied to my case, then it imposes on me a duty to try to persuade the parents to inform the daughter, or to allow me to do so. Failing this, it imposes a duty on me to do so. As a counter-argument, the parents could point out that according to their belief system, everything – including personal autonomy – is restricted by obedience to the Law of God, so disclosure could interfere with the daughter's God-given injunction to marry and be fruitful.

The implication of the above example is that it is always the parents – perhaps acting as the representatives of the religion – who make the demands that religious considerations should be paramount. That this is not so is illustrated by the case of a boy who has moderately severe spastic quadriplegic cerebral palsy, but who is intellectually able. When it came to schooling, the equipment required because of his physical limitations, and in particular the physiotherapy required to help him to overcome those limitations, was not available within the Jewish private school system, so the parents agreed that he should attend a secular school for the physically disabled. Even at the age of five, he found it impossible to settle in the school, and he was able to articulate his worries that the school was interfering with the observance of his religion. He therefore transferred to one of the Jewish schools where, although he did not receive adequate physical support, he made much better academic progress. This illustrates the over-riding need, at least in some of these children, to be within their own community from a very early age, if they are to thrive. Again, which is the greater harm? Apart from the lack of education and care to which this child is subject, there is the question of allocation of scarce resources. If support could be found that was acceptable to the school, should it be provided in the Jewish private school at the potential expense of another child within the Local Education Authority schools?

A potentially dangerous problem can arise as a result of the perceived need of many of these families for the existence of the disabled child to be kept secret. It is normal practice for the conclusions of a consultation to be passed on to the patient's general practitioner. Permission to do this is often withheld by these families. In one instance, my diagnosis of fragile X syndrome was unknown to the general practitioner, and his diagnosis of epilepsy was unknown to me. As a result, we were treating the child with mutually antagonistic drugs.

The second part of the book will consider the issues raised by the first section. First, many of the difficulties encountered in attempting to accommodate the beliefs of patients when defining their treatment arise because of the perception in liberal societies that patients' beliefs must be respected and that it is in their interest to do this. It is questionable whether in fact this is an overriding requirement, or whether there are circumstances in which beliefs must be ignored in the interest either of the patient or of other parties such as the wider host society. Secondly, and arising in part from this question of respect for beliefs, there is the question of whose interests have to be safeguarded, since the patients being considered are minors, and are often either too young or too immature to make their wishes known. Who speaks for the child, and is able to make decisions in the child's best interest? It can be questioned whether it is necessarily the parent, particularly since it is often the case that the parent is acting as the agent of the minority culture and is constrained by that culture with regard to the choices that can be made, but nevertheless the interests of the parent must be considered. Thirdly, the interests of the doctor in refraining from colluding in what he or she believes to be inappropriate treatment have to be considered and a decision made as to which should take preference – the right of patients to make autonomous decisions about their own treatment or the treatment of their children, or the professional integrity and autonomy of the doctor.

In addition to the interests of individuals, two wider interests must also be considered, namely those of the minority culture itself and those of the wider host community. This will to a large extent depend on the consideration of the relative harm caused by complying, or not, with the religious requirements. It may be necessary to accept a less effective treatment, if it maintains the family integrity. What is the balance of harm and benefit? The key phrase here is 'less effective'. It is questionable whether it could ever be justified to expect a physician or the host community to comply with ineffective or harmful treatment in order to respect the religious beliefs of the patient or their parents.

In discussing whether the interests of the minority culture should be subject to the need to comply with, say, the laws of the majority culture, special note must be taken of the fact that the main group under discussion, namely the Hasidim, may be in a unique position, since of all Jews they suffered most at the hands of the Nazis, and the vast majority of the victims of the Holocaust were from these groups. They were indeed coerced into complying with the anti-Semitic laws of Germany at that time, with appalling results. Since it could be argued that there is a debt owed to them by the Gentile community as a result of this, it has to be asked whether such groups can be expected to accept that they have duties to the majority culture, and whether this debt should influence the duties that the majority culture has to them.

In summary, therefore, the insistence by members of the groups under discussion that their religious beliefs must be paramount does raise problems both for individual doctors and for the host community. These range from complete denial of the existence of the disabled child, with implications of neglect, to insistence on collusion with inadequate therapy, or diversion of scarce resources to the group from other vulnerable groups.

The final section of this book will suggest ways in which these dilemmas may be solved. Clearly, even if they are regarded as a group with special interests within the host community, groups such as the Hasidim are members of that host community and must accept at least some of the legal and moral duties of that membership. The fact that some modification of these duties can be achieved without undue harm to the host community in order to accommodate religious belief is seen, for example, in the various allowances that are made to Sikhs in the legislation relating to protective headgear,[8,9] but nevertheless compliance with the law is required. It will be suggested that if the religious schools can be brought to a standard which complies with, say, health and safety regulations and acceptable standards of curriculum and teacher competence, then recognition of the schools for grant-aided status might be possible. This would open the way for resolution of the problem of meeting the needs of disabled children within these communities on the same terms that they are met for such children in the host community.

References

1   Jarman B (1983) Identification of underprivileged areas. *BMJ*. **286**: 1705–9.

2   Jarman B (1984) Underprivileged areas: validation and distribution of scores. *BMJ*. **289**: 1587–92.

3   London Research Centre (1997) *Focus on London 97* (edited by J Church and A Holding). The Stationery Office, London, p. 86.

4   Jimack M (1989) *Research into Hackney Jewry*. Federation of Jewish Family Services, London.

5   Dein S (1992) Letters to the Rebbe: millennium, messianism and medicine among the Lubavitch of Stamford Hill. *Int J Soc Psychiatry*. **38**: 262–72.

6   Jakobovits I (1975) *Jewish Medical Ethics*. Bloch Publishing Company, New York, p. 155.

7   Emson EH (1992) Rights, duties and responsibilities in health care. *J Appl Phil*. **9**: 3–11.

8   *Motor-Cycle Crash Helmets (Religious Exemptions) Act 1976*. HMSO, London.

9   *Employment Act 1989*. HMSO, London.

Chapter 2

Impairment, disability and handicap

In technical writing no less than in common speech, the terms 'impairment', 'disability' and 'handicap' are often used synonymously. However, differentiation between the three concepts is useful in discussing attitudes to them. In the *International Classification of Impairments, Disabilities and Handicaps*,[1] the following definitions are given.

- Impairment: *any loss or abnormality of psychological, physiological or anatomical structure or function.*
- Disability: *any restriction or lack . . . of ability to perform an activity . . . considered normal for a human being.*
- Handicap: *a disadvantage for a given individual, resulting from an impairment or a disability, that limits or prevents the fulfilment of a role that is normal (depending on age, sex, and social and cultural factors) for that individual.*[1]

An important differentiation that needs to be made is between attitudes to a defect in oneself and to defects in others, since both will influence the extent to which they are handicapping. Lansdown and Polak[2] found consistency across two countries, with pictures of children with a cleft lip or protruding teeth being most often rejected, but they found that children who themselves had had a cleft lip repaired showed no increase in overt disturbed behaviour compared with children without facial deformities. Pueschel[3] quotes Olbrisch,[4] who claimed that Down syndrome children are stigmatised by their appearance and are thought to be stupid looking. Pueschel himself found that 72% of parents were not concerned about the effect of their child's appearance, and 83% felt that the child was well accepted by society.[5]

Comparing children who have facial deformity with controls without such deformity, Lansdown *et al.*[6] found that the more severely deformed children appeared to adjust best. They suggested that these children expect negative responses to such an extent that they are not surprised or upset by them, whereas the less severely deformed do not receive such a consistently negative response, and are therefore often anxious about what the response will be. On the other hand, observers considered that the children whom they rated as more attractive would be happier, more clever, more friendly and easier to get along with.[6]

This emphasises the fact that what constitutes an impairment to one person may not necessarily seem to be a problem to another. In the television programme *Your Life in Their Hands*, people sought cosmetic plastic surgery for what was for them a damagingly misshapen nose or ear, correction of which appeared to increase their confidence and sense of well-being, even though the surgeon had had to make a wire silhouette of the original nose in order to convince them of the change.[7]

Attitudes to impairment and disability are coloured by the concept of normality – that is, the requirement to conform to what is usual for the majority, or what is considered desirable within the wider community. Oliver has attacked the claim that the abilities of the majority (e.g. the ability to walk) are something to which the disabled should aspire, or should be taught to aspire. He objected to the two underlying assumptions, namely that the main aim of the non-walker is to walk, and that they cannot do this because they lack the will to walk.[8] A subsidiary point that can be made here in support of Oliver is that people often fail to realise that an impairment that would constitute a major disability for the majority who do not have it, is much less disabling (if at all) to those who have lived with it for a long time, or for the whole of their lives. Oliver also claims that normality cannot be achieved because it does not exist. In fact, he seems to be implying something else, namely that norms exist, but that no two people have the same norms. Clearly, he cannot here be referring to statistical norms, but instead to what the individual regards as desirable or ideal. To support this, he quotes Ladd (answering a question from the floor at an international conference), who claimed that although for parents the birth of a deaf child might be a tragedy, for the deaf community it is a precious gift, since for the deaf community it is normal to be deaf. On a slightly different point – that the ideal for a group may not be attainable even for those who are within the group – he refers to the Nazi belief that the Aryan ideal should have blond hair and blue eyes, even though many fervent and accepted Nazis (including Adolf Hitler) did not conform to the ideal.

The original definitions of disability and handicap refer to 'normal for a human being' and 'normal for that individual'. Although the latter definition takes into account age, sex and cultural factors, it seems unlikely that the cultural group of, say, the deaf is being referred to. Yet such a group is a cultural unit, with as predictable a response to those who do not conform to the group norms as any other group. For example, individuals with Usher syndrome, who grow up in the deaf community until they start to go blind in their late teens, then begin to feel excluded. There is a deaf community where, although the deaf child has an impairment, she is at no social disadvantage. Only when she has to cope in the hearing community is she disadvantaged because of their inability to communicate with her. Even here, however, *both* are handicapped – the deaf child by the hearing person's inability to understand signs, and the hearing person by the deaf child's inability to understand speech. This is directly equivalent to two people, neither of whom speaks the other's language, trying to communicate with each other. Neither is handicapped except in that very specific situation, and each is then equally handicapped. However, this is not entirely straightforward, since the deaf community is the minority and its members have to function within the majority hearing community in order to acquire the necessities of daily life, whereas most members of the majority culture may never have to communicate with a deaf person.

The handicapping effect of labelling, and the tendency of the medical profession, paramedical professions and even the public at large to view people with disabilities as lifelong patients who are in need of treatment, are also important. Brisenden's main thrust is against the tendency to define people by their diagnosis (e.g. the cerebrally palsied, the mentally retarded), but he goes further than this, by questioning the use of jargon which has a quite different meaning for the laity and the professional. He mentions the term 'spastic' which, with reason, he claims conjures up visions of a drooling idiot, although technically it only implies a form of muscle stiffness, as well as the generalisation 'the disabled'. He points out that an antonym for 'disabled' is 'normal', for which another antonym is 'abnormal'. Such labelling is handicapping not only because it is demeaning, but also because it enables not only the needs of the person with the disability to be forgotten, but also the fact that they are a person at all, capable of assessing and articulating their own needs.[9] He points out that in 'Physical disability in 1986 and beyond: a report of the Royal College of Physicians', the needs of disabled people are viewed entirely in terms of their *medical* needs, and that it recommends the setting up of regional Disability Centres based in District General Hospitals.[10] Although he is not entirely fair, in that the report is concerned mainly with the medical needs of disabled people, he makes the fair point that no disabled people appear to have been consulted when preparing the report, and that the latter does refer throughout to 'patients'.

The tendency to take a rather narrow view of the needs and abilities of people with disabilities is illustrated by the decision of the United States Supreme Court that a deaf woman was not improperly excluded from a nurse training programme, since the reason was not her disability as such, but the fact that this disability made it impossible for her to do the job safely. Joe has pointed out that no account was taken of the many deaf healthcare professionals who are already working, or of the plaintiff's strengths or ability to cope with modification of the curriculum. The court concentrated only on situations where the impairment could endanger patients, and not on those areas where the woman could perform safely. He suggests that a handicap must be described in terms of 'the specific functional capacities and limitations an individual brings to a particular situation', if discrimination is to be eliminated.[11]

The truth of this relativity of handicap can be seen most vividly in fiction. HG Wells, in his short story *The Country of the Blind*, turns the usual situation on its head. A sighted mountaineer arrives in a valley that has been completely cut off from the outside world for generations and where, as a result of inbreeding, all of the inhabitants are born without eyes. Initially he sees this as a godsend, since 'in the country of the blind the one-eyed man is king'. However, what becomes apparent is not only his own abnormality in this environment, but also the fact that he is regarded as unformed, and almost sub-human, by the community, such that when he falls in love with his master's daughter, the only solution is to make him normal by surgically removing his eyes.[12]

The above example is drawn from fiction, but it is mirrored in real life by the belief that the odd one out must not only conform to majority norms, but would actually want to do so because it would be good for him or her. Again it is assumed that the able know best what is good for the disabled person. This is seen, for example, in the oral tradition of teaching the deaf, which at its extreme forbids any form of signing on the grounds that the child will become dependent on the signs and never learn to speak. In children who are so profoundly deaf that they are incapable of learning speech, this not only prevents them from communicating with their deaf and hearing peers at the time, but it also interferes with the flowering of their innate language, putting them at a lifelong disadvantage.

The same feature can be seen if we consider not disability itself but the related concept of disease. Disease is defined as an 'unhealthy condition of body or mind, or some part thereof; illness, sickness; particular kind of this with special symptoms or location'.[13] Thus in the biomedical model of disease the patient presents with complaints (symptoms), and the doctor defines abnormalities of clinical examination or investigation (signs), which leads to a differential diagnosis. This can be refined by further examination to give a firm diagnosis. Treatment can then be instituted which aims to alleviate the symptoms and at best the signs as well.

As an example, I wish to consider non-organic or hysterical visual loss, a condition that can be analysed according to the above model, but which has an effect on different patients which ranges from the extremely damaging, through complete neutrality to the frankly beneficial. It mirrors disability and handicap, since the same impairment can have different effects on different people at different times. I shall describe a series of patients with the condition, and then discuss whether any or all of them have a disease, and if so, how this can be defined.

Hysteria is the presence of signs and symptoms in the absence of physical abnormality sufficient to cause them, conforming to the patient's concept of disease rather than to anatomy, physiology or pathology, the whole being viewed as a means of escaping from a stressful life situation. In some patients such stress is not apparent, and the concept of the sick role is brought into play, the suggestion being that the extra attention afforded to the sick fulfils an emotional need in the patient.[14]

Patient A presented at 29 years of age with severe restriction of her visual fields and severely diminished visual acuity of 20 years' standing. This was restricting her so much that she was housebound unless she was accompanied. After it had been explained to her that her eyes were healthy and her symptoms were the result of stress, she was able to discuss in detail the longstanding sexual abuse that she had suffered between the ages of 9 and 16 years. Her vision improved and she was able to get a job. The symptoms recurred four years later, and she attributed this to the media attention that was paid to sexual abuse at that time.

Patient B presented with blurred vision and difficulty in coping at school. She was a small child, not academically able, and poor at sports. Despite the fact that investigations were entirely normal and her vision returned within days of the explanation, the parents did not accept the diagnosis. One month later, patient B presented to another hospital with an hysterical limp.

Patient C presented at the age of 9 years having failed a school eye test. She then complained of difficulty in seeing the blackboard, and she was having academic problems. She had diminished vision and restricted fields. After an explanation had been given to her and the school, the symptoms resolved.

Patient D also failed a school eye test, and had similar signs to patient C. However, she had no symptoms whatsoever, and the signs resolved spontaneously.

Patient E presented at the age of 10 years with diminished vision and constricted fields. Investigation was entirely normal. After 12 years there has been no alteration in the signs. From childhood, patient E had wanted to be a nurse, but she was academically unable to do this. She leads a full life, and appears to be happy in her job. The symptoms are only present in two situations – when she is being tested by a doctor, and when she needs an explanation for why she did not become a nurse.

How are we to understand the idea of disease appearing in these examples? Boorse describes 'the crucial element in the idea of a biological design, the notion of a natural function'. He states 'that the single unifying property of all recognised diseases of plants and animals appears to be this: that they interfere with one or more functions typically performed within members of the species'.[15] Although he does not actually discuss vision, we can say that since good vision would conform to 'the natural design of the organism', all of the above patients are diseased, in that in none of them is the visual system performing 'naturally'. Indeed, they can all be said to have the same disease. Moreover, since his definition of health is to be free of disease, none of them can be said to be healthy, since health 'consists in the performance of each part of its natural function'.

However, we can take a wider view of health, such as that held by Katherine Mansfield: 'By health I mean the power to live a full, adult, living, breathing life . . . I want to be all that I am capable of becoming'.[16]

According to this view, for patient D the state of her eyes – natural or not – is unimportant, and for patient E it could be argued that only by *having* the abnormal findings can she come anywhere near to fulfilling the requirements of such a definition, since it allows her to live a full adult life, being all that she is in fact capable of becoming.

Since the condition is essential for patient E's health, and health has been defined by Boorse as the absence of disease, is hysterical visual loss by this definition a disease? Boorse goes some way towards resolving this by distinguishing between disease and illness – an illness being a disease of sufficient severity to incapacitate – and he does cite instances of disease being beneficial (e.g. flat feet in the reluctant draftee).[15] However, this example does not meet the need, since we are discussing here not the use of coincident pathology to avoid an unpleasant situation, but abnormal findings arising from the stress itself. Boorse derives two definitions of health, namely the absence of disease and the absence of illness. According to Boorse, an illness must be a reasonably serious disease with incapacitating effects which make it undesirable. By both of these definitions, since sight is affected, the eyes are not performing their natural function, they are therefore diseased, and patient E is not healthy. However, since patient E's life is in no way impaired by the lack of function, she suffers no incapacitating effects from it, and her life is indeed enhanced by it. We might argue then that she has no illness and is therefore healthy. However, patient A does meet Boorse's criterion for an illness, since she was completely incapacitated by the symptoms and could only return to normal function when they had resolved. It thus appears that one can say that the same clinical condition is a disease in all of its manifestations, since it represents a failure of natural function, but nevertheless it is an illness in one context but not in another. Sacks makes a similar point when discussing two patients with temporal lobe epilepsy which manifested as reminiscences. In the case of one patient who was assailed by a cacophony of half-remembered tunes, this disrupted her life, but in the other patient the memories of a lost childhood were healing: 'Mrs O'C declined anticonvulsants: 'I *need* these memories', she would say . . . Thus she felt her illness as health, as *healing*'.[17]

However, there is a further complication to Boorse's account of illness and disease. In attempting to overcome the statistics that would, for example, make tooth decay normal, Boorse claims that disturbed function becomes unnatural, and therefore disease, if it is either atypical for the species or is mainly due to hostile environmental factors.[15] How does this addition bear on our patients? In all but patient D there are clear hostile interferences in the environment (failure to achieve academic expectations in cases B, C and E, failure of the parents to come to terms with this in case B, and sexual abuse in case A). Yet can they be said to have caused the visual loss in the same way that food residues cause tooth decay, or should the whole complex be seen as lying outside the realm of medicine? Is this just another example of cultural iatrogenesis, and are we, as Illich claims, just undermining the client's ability to come to terms with reality?[18] The child comes to the attention of the medical profession because of the assumption that there is something wrong with their eyes that is causing the visual loss, and hopefully it is something amenable to treatment. Once it is established that this is not so, it may be that medicine has no further part to play other than reassurance and dismissal. Boorse goes some way towards acknowledging this in that his definition of illness is evaluative, as different people will find different levels of interference with function incapacitating. Indeed, the same person may find the same level of interference incapacitating in one situation but not in another.

Since we have accepted that the hysterical visual loss can be a means of coping with stress, it can in fact be viewed as a health-promoting device. Clearly it is easiest to make this case with regard to patient E, and perhaps most difficult for patient D, since in the latter there appears to be no interference with health anyway. This is perhaps best borne out by patient B, since 'curing' the visual loss necessitated the development of another coping mechanism, namely a limp. If the visual loss is regarded as a health-promoting device rather than a disease, what is it promoting? Greaves[19] suggests that seeking epidemiological factors to explain cot death, for example, locks us into the medical model with its insistence on finding a pathological explanation. I would suggest that in seeking epidemiological factors in hysteria, we should be seeking not the aetiology of hysteria (since this is in fact the stress), but the aetiology of the disease itself – the stress that requires the hysteria for its control. This is saying more than that the visual loss is only a symptom, and is no more health promoting than the pain of appendicitis, serving only to draw attention to the underlying disease. It is a claim that health and disease can coexist, in that if the person can produce coping strategies, then they can be healthy even if a part of them is not. Health becomes a matter of overall positive balance. Sade sums this up as follows: 'health should be understood as the condition of a living thing whose biological functions are operating in a way that promotes uncompromised living, holding the organism's flourishing life as the standard . . . one can speak of body parts . . . as being healthy or not, but the idea of health . . . applies to the whole person'.[20] Here health is therefore defined as not merely the absence of life-threatening disease, but also the ability to be free of those conditions that interfere with a flourishing life. He cites the case of the 70-year-old with a lifelong disfigurement which has prevented social intercourse, whose life is not threatened, but who is nevertheless not flourishing, and therefore could be said to be unhealthy. A healthy person is therefore one who has an overall strategy for coping with life – who is a whole person. However, there does have to be an overall positive balance. Patient A, despite having developed what I am suggesting amounts to a coping strategy, was still functionally disabled. In that it is rarely possible to remove the stress, a person can only be described as healthy if their coping strategy is adequate. In patient A this was certainly not so – indeed it was adding to the stress and thus to the disease process.

Therefore the role of the doctor in a condition such as hysterical visual loss is not to remove the visual loss *per se*, but to assist the patient in doing so in a way that sets in its place a greater ability to face the reality of their situation – the reverse of Illich's cultural iatrogenesis.

I am suggesting that health should be understood in the context of a condition such as hysterical visual loss as a state of balance in which the whole person can cope with life, disease should be understood as any process that precipitates the need for coping strategies and illness should be viewed as the failure to produce such strategies adequately. On this basis, patients A and B are ill, patients C and E are diseased but healthy, and patient D, so far as one can tell, is neither diseased nor ill. Can this be generalised? Greer *et al.*[21] have shown that patients with breast cancer who deny the seriousness of the condition, far from doing badly, have among the most favourable prognoses. In a letter reporting a 15-year follow-up,[22] they were able to show that 45% of those who had responded to the cancer with denial or a fighting spirit were still alive and free of recurrence, compared with only 17% of those whose responded with fatalism or helplessness. When all other prognostic factors were examined individually, psychological response was found to be the most important factor in determining death of these patients from any cause (not just death from the cancer itself), and also the time of first recurrence of the cancer. According to my hypothesis, the denial would act as a coping strategy sufficient to inhibit even this most biological of conditions.

It is perhaps a cliché to say that health and illness are functions of the whole person, but it is less obvious that disease is, too. The implications of this are that even the most apparently local disease must be treated within the whole, and also that much which appears to be disease, even obviously biological disease, may not be the exclusive province of the doctor. Applying the above discussion of disease to our original subject, namely disability and handicap, the normality or abnormality of the individual is a function of their whole functioning, not merely of the effect of the impairment.

Hare,[23] in an attempt to define health and distinguish it from disease, takes this further. He points out that whether a thing is a disease or an illness, a disability or a handicap, depends to a large extent on the person in whom it occurs and the society in which it occurs. He describes a South American tribe in which dyschromic spirochaetosis is almost universal, and consequently the coloured skin lesions which it induces are regarded as so desirable that those few members of the tribe who escape the infection are unable to obtain marriage partners. The question then arises as to whether this is a disease in the tribe, or only if it is caught by strangers. In attempting to understand the controversy over the concept of disease and illness, he produces the following general formula:

> *A exhibits observable features F . . . F*
> *So A has condition C*
> *But C is a disease*
> *So A is not healthy*
> *But T is the treatment most likely to remove C*
> *So A ought to be given T.*[23]

This seems to be an acceptable scheme apart from one thing. Who decides that condition C is a disease? If C is malaria, then the scheme fits the mainstream of orthodox medicine. However, if C is political deviance and T is incarceration in an asylum, or C is homosexuality, then it does not – the decision that these conditions are diseases being political and social, rather than medical. Hare suggests that if the patient feels that C is bad for him then it is a disease, so that malaria is a disease, political deviance is not, and homosexuality may be – depending on the subject's attitude to it. However, even this is not straightforward, since the homosexual's attitude will be conditioned by the culture in which he has grown up, and social conditioning can make a political deviant believe that he is diseased. This was the conclusion, for example, of George Orwell's *1984*.[24] This can to some extent be applied to disability and handicap, since we are culturally conditioned in our responses to groups different from our own. If C is defined by the hearing community, for example, as the inability of the deaf to communicate in the hearing world, then lack of speech is a handicap, and T consists of teaching the deaf to speak. However, if C is defined by the deaf community as the inability of the hearing to communicate in the deaf world, then the lack of signing is a handicap, and T consists of teaching the hearing to sign.

Labels that are used to differentiate groups which are different from our own may be detrimental, but as Sade[20] has pointed out, labelling a thing as a disease or a disability can have positive as well as negative effects. For example, labelling alcoholism or compulsive gambling as a disease rather than as delinquency results in those who have the problem receiving sympathy and help, whereas labelling homosexuality in this way has the negative effect of making homosexuals appear to be abnormal, sick individuals who are in need of treatment.

Hutchison[25] has attempted to unify the medical and social models. He defines the following six concepts:

- A: disease, disorder or damage
- B: loss or abnormality of function due to A
- C: restriction of expected activity due to A or B
- D: prevention of fulfilment of expected social roles due to B or C
- E: prevention of fulfilment of expected social roles due to F
- F: social structure, attitudes and resources – related to A.

Hutchison points out that the medical model runs from A (the disorder) to B (the impairment) to C (the disability) to D (the handicap), but largely ignores E and F. On the other hand, in the social model the person is central, being acted upon in one direction by the disorder A, resulting in the impairment B, and in the other direction by the social environment F, resulting in the disability E.

In his combined model, Hutchison has two complementary sequences, and again the person is central. In the first sequence, condition A, through impairment B to disability C, and environment F, through discrimination E to disadvantage D acts on the person in a negative way. On the other hand, an identical sequence can be built up consisting of condition A, through strength B to ability C, and environment F through privilege E to advantage D, emphasising the positive aspects. It is surprising that this concept appears so innovative, since it should be the basis of all treatment programmes for people who are disabled. The person's strengths must be the starting point for treatment, since only by knowing what they can already do can one plan ways of helping them to do more. This offers a model for analysing the needs of, say, a population within and without the Hasidic community, since it forces not only a consideration of the disadvantages for the child and for the wider community of conforming to the tenets of strict religious belief, but also a consideration of the strengths that belonging to the community bring to the child and his or her family, and the effect that potentially has in relieving the demands for wider services. Again, by placing the disabled person at the centre, with the disadvantages of the impairment being counterbalanced by the strengths of the person and their cultural environment, it forces a consideration of the wishes of the person involved – of what they see as a life that is normal for them, rather than the 'normalisation' which is required by society at large.

In summary, whether one is considering impairment, disability and handicap, or health, disease and illness, decisions about what falls within each of these categories have an evaluative element. What constitutes any one of the categories depends on the person to whom it occurs, will vary for that person over time, and will depend on the ambient culture.

References

1 World Health Organization (1980) *International Classification of Impairments, Disabilities and Handicaps*. World Health Organization, Geneva, pp. 27, 28, 29.

2 Lansdown R and Polak L (1975) A study of the psychological effects of facial deformity in children. *Child Care Health Dev.* **1**: 85–91.

3 Pueschel SM (1988) Facial plastic surgery for children with Down syndrome. *Dev Med Child Neurol.* **30**: 540–3.

4 Olbrisch RR (1982) Plastic surgical management of children with Down syndrome: indications and results. *Br J Plastic Surg.* **35**: 195–200.

5 Pueschel SM, Monteiro LA and Erickson M (1986) Parents' and physicians' perceptions of facial plastic surgery in children with Down syndrome. *J Ment Defic Res.* **30**: 71–9.

6 Lansdown R, Lloyd J and Hunter J (1991) Facial deformity in childhood: severity and psychological adjustment. *Child Care Health Dev.* **17**: 165–71.

7 BBC Television (1991) *Your Life in Their Hands. Striving for perfection?* Broadcast on 10 May.

8 Oliver M (1989) Conductive education: if it wasn't so sad it would be funny. *Disabil Handicap Soc.* **4**: 197–200.

9 Brisenden S (1986) Independent living and the medical model of disability. *Disabil Handicap Soc.* **1**: 173–8.

10 Brisenden S (1987) A response to physical disability in 1986 and beyond: a report of the Royal College of Physicians. *Disabil Handicap Soc.* **2**: 175–82.

11 Joe TC (1981) Rethinking the concept of 'handicapped'. *Arch Phys Med Rehabil.* **62**: 236–8.

12 Wells HG (1967) The country of the blind. Reprinted in: C Dolley (ed.) *The Penguin Book of English Short Stories.* Penguin Books, Harmondsworth, p. 110.

13 Sykes JB (ed.) (1976) *Concise Oxford Dictionary* (6e). Oxford University Press, Oxford.

14 Jones RB and Levy IS (1983) Hysterical blindness. In: K Wybar and D Taylor (eds) *Pediatric Ophthalmology. Current aspects.* Marcel Dekker Inc., New York, pp. 399–406.

15 Boorse C (1981) On the distinction between disease and illness. In: M Cohen, T Nagel and T Scanlon (eds) *Medicine and Moral Philosophy.* Princeton University Press, Princeton, NJ, pp. 3–22.

16 Stead CK (ed.) (1977) *The Letters and Journals of Katherine Mansfield.* Penguin Books, Harmondsworth, p. 278.

17 Sacks O (1986) *The Man Who Mistook His Wife for a Hat.* Picador, London, p. 137.

18 Illich I (1976) *Limits to Medicine.* Penguin Books, Harmondsworth, p. 133.

19 Greaves D (1988) Sudden infant deaths: models of health and illness. *J Appl Phil.* **5**: 61–74.

20 Sade RM (1995) A theory of health and disease: the objectivist–subjectivist dichotomy. *J Med Phil.* **20**: 513–25.

21 Greer S, Morris T and Pettingale KW (1979) Psychological response to breast cancer: effect on outcome. *Lancet.* **2**: 785–7.

22 Greer S, Morris T, Pettingale KW and Haybittle JL (1990) Psychological response to breast cancer and 15-year outcome. *Lancet.* **335**: 49–50.

23 Hare RM (1986) Health. *J Med Ethics.* **12**: 174–81.

24 Orwell G (1949) *1984.* Secker & Warburg, London.

25 Hutchison T (1995) The classification of disability. *Arch Dis Child.* **73**: 91–3.

Chapter 3

Cultural attitudes to disability

The way in which adherents of a religion respond to disability and illness, or even the way in which they are manifested, will depend not only on the teachings of the religion, but also on education, national identity, level of affluence and so on, as well as on how strictly the religion is followed. Studies comparing different religious groups are often not clear whether the religious affiliation is active or not. For example, the majority of people in the UK will appear, from their hospital records, to be 'C of E' (Church of England). Thus, for example, if a comparison was made of the attitudes to disability shown by a group of devout Hasidic Jews and a matched group of Anglicans whose only evidence of religious practice was derived from the hospital records, then like would not be being compared with like, and any conclusions about the different responses of the adherents of the two religions to disability would be invalid.

As well as the attitudes to disability as embodied in the religion, one must also consider the social attitudes of families to their disabled offspring, partly arising from perceived stigma in the community. In a study of attitudes to cerebral palsy among different immigrant groups in Israel, Mundel comments that one mother complained after treatment had resulted in three of her children who had previously been immobile becoming mobile.[1] From her perspective, what would be considered by most people to be a major improvement was for her a disaster, since it deprived her of the means that she had used to conceal her shame and guilt.

This is also illustrated by the case of a child of Hasidic Jewish parents who had Down syndrome, and whose parents' plan was, in the mother's own words, 'To hide her as long as possible'. There are two main reasons for this stance. First, the presence of a congenitally disabled person in the family is regarded as a disgrace in that it may, for example, imply that he or she was conceived during a forbidden period of the menstrual cycle, and therefore resulted from the mother's failure to comply with the religious law. Secondly, since in this culture marriages are arranged within quite small groups, families with a history of disability may have difficulty in finding partners for the other children in the family. Wieselberg points out that this is a potent motive for not acknowledging the presence of a disabled individual in these families.[2] Furthermore, it may lead to estrangement within the wider family if the same constraints are brought to bear on them.

Similarly, in another example a child was never acknowledged by his family, his siblings were not allowed to play with him, and they were not told that he was their brother. In effect this family was going even further and denying even within the immediate family that their own child was a member of that family. It is interesting that Mundel found in immigrant families in Israel that mothers when counting their children often left out the disabled child as if he or she did not exist.[1]

It is tempting to regard any response to disability within a community as if it were specific to that community, whereas of course it may be a more general response. The belief that all children should be perfect, and that they can be made so, exacerbates the effect on the family of a disabled child in all cultures.

It must also be remembered that, for example, Jewishness is not the only attribute of a person who is Jewish. In a cross-cultural study of attitudes to surgically correctable birth defects such as cleft palate, Strauss found that among Israeli Jews attitudes tended to vary according to country of origin.[3] Oriental Jews tended to have a fatalistic explanation, with those from Iraq regarding it as a punishment for past sins in the family, and therefore a stigma on the family, whereas those from Morocco or the Yemen viewing it as an indiscriminate act of God and therefore not a stigma. Western Jews, on the other hand, interpreted disability in medical terms and expected much of medicine. Strauss points out that although it is tempting (and possibly correct) to see this difference in cultural terms, Western Jews are in general much more highly educated than Oriental Jews, and there is a strong correlation between level of education and attitudes to disability and its aetiology.[3] Mundel also found variation among the immigrant groups from North Africa, who all tended to have a fatalistic view of disability, but some of whom treated the disabled person with acceptance and mercy, while others displayed attitudes of social rejection and guilt.[1]

Despite this acknowledged difference in both studies between the Middle Eastern groups and the European groups, members of all groups sought religious help, in particular undertaking pilgrimages and consulting rabbis and wise men. Dein, in a study of the Lubavitch,[4] comments on the role of the Rebbe as healer. He points out that illness or disability is seen as resulting from spiritual disorder, and many write to the Rebbe seeking his advice. The reply usually defines the religious disorder which, it is claimed, accounts for the illness, and which when corrected results in near-miraculous cure. The fault is often said to be in the Mezuzot (the ritual scrolls placed on doorposts to protect the house and its inmates from harm). Dein cites the case of a man who suffered a heart attack. The Rebbe's response was that the Mezuzot were not kosher. Sure enough, the word 'heart' was mis-spelt in the scroll.[4]

Wieselberg also comments on the role of the Rebbe when she describes her practice of structural family therapy with ultra-orthodox families.[2] One young married couple was experiencing difficulty in being accepted as adoptive parents because the husband had not come to terms with their infertility, despite the fact that the wife had a congenitally absent uterus. They had been told by the Rebbe that prayer would result in them being given a baby. She explained this as the baby being granted to them by adoption rather than by miracle, thus allowing the husband to accept the infertility without doubting the Rebbe.[2]

On the other hand, if the disability is accepted, Hasidic families are keen to ensure that the children receive all of the medical help that is necessary. For example, in a study of immunisation uptake, Cuninghame *et al.* found no significant difference between Hasidic families and the rest of the inhabitants of the borough.[5] Law and Wallfish compared a group of Hasidic children with a group of Gentile children in the use of speech therapy services.[6] They found that uptake was good, with far more Jewish families than Gentile families keeping the first appointment.

However, therapy is only taken up within the terms of reference of the community, and this may have a bearing on the role of the therapist. For example, in outlining the problems encountered by a secular psycho-therapist working with a mentally disturbed ultra-orthodox young man, Bilu and Witztum emphasise the role played by the patient's perception of the therapist.[7] They point out that 'the fact that the secular unabash-edly breach the religious commandments viewed by the observant as the sine qua non of Jewish life makes contacts with them in many spheres of life virtually impossible'. Given that the spiritual ideal for the ultra-orthodox Jew is the strict fulfilment of the Law and the study of the sacred texts, with religion thus embracing all aspects of their life, it would be expected that their understanding of the causation of illness and the vocabulary used to express their symptoms and distress would reflect this. Bilu and Witztum describe the case of a young man with a depressive psychosis who believed that his behaviour was dictated by visitations from an angel, whom he conjured up with a ceremony involving candles placed in a particular geometric configuration.[7] By taking part in this ceremony with his Rabbi, they were able to exorcise the angel and bring about a marked improvement in his condition.

Although they claim that this is culturally sensitive therapy, it does highlight the question of collusion of the therapist with the patient's delusion. On the other hand, Wieselberg was able to show that, as an orthodox Jew herself, once she had been accepted by the family as a therapist she was able to use the ritual and respect for authority that is inherent in Judaism as a positive therapeutic tool to help the family.[2] She makes the point that these families would often prefer to be treated by a Gentile than by a non-practising Jew.

Cross-cultural disorders may involve culturally specific symptoms. In order to analyse the effect of the religious belief of the patient on the manifestation of a disease or disability, I have chosen obsessive-compulsive disorder, since it would seem probable that the insistence on ritual that is a feature of many religions could well manifest itself in this disorder. Greenberg and Witztum found in Israel that among an ultra-orthodox population, although this disorder was no more common than among secular Jews, the symptomatology was often determined by the religion.[8] Those areas in which an intense ritual is required in any case (e.g. cleansing after menstruation, ablutions before prayers, or the strict separation of milk and meat) commonly became compulsive obsessions in those with the disorder. It is interesting that although the Shulkhan Arukh (the code of Jewish law which governs every minute aspect of life for an ultra-orthodox Jew) can itself border on the obsessive, patients and their families have no difficulty in recognising a pathological extension of this, and indeed had often sought help from Rabbis before coming to see the therapist.[8] Goshen-Gottstein also comments that Rabbis in a religious college will often note if, for example, ritual hand-washing in a particular student exceeds that required by strict adherence to the Law, and will then seek help for him.[9] Greenberg and Witztum conclude that 'if the religious setting is ignored, the excessive concerns with dirt, orderliness, aggression and sex, and the compulsive behaviours of washing, repeating, checking and slowness are typical of obsessive-compulsive disorder',[8] so that – as might be expected – the culture determines the direction of the disorder but does not precipitate it.[8] This view is supported by Riddle *et al.*[10] who, when defining the phenomenology in a group of children and adolescents with obsessive-compulsive disorder attending their clinic, found that obsessive attention to ritual, washing, sexual thoughts and contamination with excreta was common. Their group was composed largely of middle-class Caucasian children. Swedo *et al.*, reporting from a similar clinic, described similar findings with similar phenomenology.[11]

Akhtar *et al.*, reporting on a similar group from India, found a virtually identical phenomenology, in particular a great concern about cleanliness and contamination with human excreta.[12] They comment that the

Hindu scriptures 'regard the human body as basically dirty and an object of disgust, and the need for repeated cleansing of the body is over-emphasised'. They also point out that 'celebration in many Indian festivals consists of bathing in a certain way or at a certain place'.[12] They make one interesting comment, namely that the paucity of sexual and religious obsessions in their group reflects 'the fact that both religion and sex are subject in India to strong social taboos . . . and that the same subtle but forceful influences that eliminate these subjects from "decent" conversation eliminate them also from overt psycho-pathology'.[12] Khanna and Channabasavanna suggest that the higher incidence of sexual and religious obsessions in their later study is evidence of changing social mores in India.[13] However, although the taboo with regard to talking about sex in the ultra-orthodox Jewish community is at least as strong, sexual obsessions occur frequently. In two Muslim communities the pattern was found to be similar. Mahgoub and Abdel-Hafeiz found that 50% of their sample presented with religious obsessions, mainly centred around Al-Woodo (the ritual washing before prayer).[14] Okasha *et al.* briefly mention that ritual washing was common in their patients with obsessive-compulsive disorder in Egypt.[15]

Scrupulosity, with excessive attention to the minutiae of religious observance, has been recognised by religious authorities from the earliest times as being pathological. Weisner and Riffel[16] and Fallon *et al.*[17] describe how this is manifested among Roman Catholic children and adolescents as over-attention to small details, such as repeatedly having to confess the same sins in order to ensure that they have been properly understood by the priest. Most of the patients had other symptoms of obsessive-compulsive disorder, and again it seems to be a case of the religion leading the symptomatology rather than causing the disease.

Goshen-Gottstein implies that, among ultra-orthodox Jews, aspects of the lifestyle, particularly the low level of concern about emotional rather than cognitive development in the community, the strict separation of the sexes from an early age, and the shame and secrecy surrounding sexual activity, puts stresses on members of the community which will tend to induce psychiatric problems.[9] However, she adduces no evidence that these problems are more common in what she describes as a religious repressive ethic.[9] In fact it would be difficult to show this, due to the impossibility of knowing the numbers living in such a community – for even if they were prepared to comply with census requirements, they are not usually sampled as a specific group.

It may not be true that religion never influences the manifestation of disease. Zylbermann *et al.* studied four groups in Israel, consisting of boys and girls in general, non-religious schools and in Orthodox religious schools. They found that in both groups of girls, and in the boys from general schools, the proportion who were short-sighted was similar to that found in other population studies, whereas among the boys in the Orthodox schools it was about three times the expected rate. They suggest that this might result from the study habits of this group, which consist of long hours of close work, associated with rhythmic rocking which causes continual alteration of the eye's focus, which they postulate could induce myopia.[18]

Behaviours that appear to be pathological may have a logical explanation if religion is taken into consideration. Charnes and Moore point out that although visiting the sick is both a religious duty and a blessing for Jews, the strictures that are placed on how far it is permitted to walk on the Sabbath may prevent such visiting, even if the patient is a child, and even if not visiting causes distress.[19] This may account for the apparent refusal to comply with treatment by insisting on taking the child out of hospital before the Sabbath begins.

The acceptance of a disabled child within a family can be a problem, and this may be influenced by the religious affiliation of the parents. Zuk examined how the acceptance of a mentally retarded child, as assessed by an interview conducted by a psychiatric social worker with the mother, was influenced by the religious affiliation of the family.[20] He found that of 27 Protestant families, 23 had problems accepting the child, as did all nine of the Jewish families, whereas 25 out of 39 Catholic families had no difficulty with acceptance. He attributes this finding to the unrelieved feelings of guilt among the Protestants and Jews. In contrast, in Catholic teaching, not only is every child regarded as a gift from God, but also it is believed that absolution from sin helps the parents to absolve themselves from guilt and therefore from the need to search their conscience for past sins that are being paid for by their having a disabled child. In the Protestant and Jewish traditions, on the other hand, the question 'What have I done to deserve a child like this?' is no less easy to answer, but there is no straightforward way of coping with the answer.[20] However, in a later paper Zuk does state that these findings are not clear-cut, and he quotes other studies in which the reverse situation has been found.[21] Boles found that for mothers of children with cerebral palsy, there was no difference in the level of anxiety among Catholic and Jewish mothers, but that this anxiety was greater than in Protestant mothers.[22] He also found that the level of guilt feelings among Catholic mothers was considerably higher than that among Jewish mothers. He reported that Catholic mothers tended to have more unrealistic attitudes towards their children than did the Jewish mothers, and also tended to be more socially withdrawn, whereas Protestant mothers were less socially withdrawn than mothers in either of the other two groups. The parents were asked about causation, and 25% agreed that it was God's punishment for having broken one of the Ten Commandments.[22] Zuk *et al.* also conducted a questionnaire study to assess acceptance of retarded children by their parents. They found that the Catholic mothers had a more intense attitude towards their religious practices than did the Protestant and Jewish mothers, and that there was a direct relationship between the intensity of religious practice and acceptance of the child.[23] Zuk *et al.* again claim that Catholic mothers are more accepting because Catholic doctrine absolves them from the guilt of having somehow caused the child's condition. Presumably this question could only be properly resolved if three groups, consisting of Catholics, Protestants and Jews, respectively, of equal size and religious intensity were compared, and Zuk and his colleagues have clearly not found such a sample.

Although they too have not found such a sample, Leyser and Dekel have reported on a religiously intense ultra-orthodox Jewish community in Israel.[24] Using an interview and rating technique, they looked at 82 families, mainly large families with up to 16 children, and almost all stable families with two married parents, whose fathers were almost all either religious students or teachers. The level of poverty was high, and the level of secular education (particularly among the mothers) was low. They estimated that about 50% of these families had made a good adjustment to the disabled child, and only about 17% had made no adjustment. The adjustment was better among younger mothers and in larger families. None of them had any contact with parent support groups. Many families felt stigmatised by the community. As they comment, it is difficult to know whether the good adjustment and low level of major problems relates to their religious belief, or to their low socio-economic status, which is known to be associated with lack of adjustment problems.[24]

In a study of the use of health services by mothers in an inner city, Watson looked at three groups: an indigenous group of Caucasian families who had been established in London for at least two generations, a group of English-speaking immigrants from various ethnic groups, and a non-English-speaking immigrant group which was entirely composed of Bengalis from Sylhet.[25] She found that although all of the groups used the services, 'the Bengalis are hampered by their lack of knowledge of what is considered good child health practice in this country'. She comments on their expectation that they will be given medicine at each visit, and their poor understanding of the difference between healthcare surveillance and treatment.[25] Why should this be so? They are a more homogeneous group than the other two groups. They all originate from a small area of Bangladesh, Sylhet, and virtually all marriages are from within this community – indeed, many are from within the same family. Although many of the mothers were born in Bangladesh, this is not universally the case, so that some of them at least will have a lifetime of experience of this country. They are Muslims who adhere strictly to the faith, particularly with regard to what is seen as the position of women in society, so that there is very little opportunity for the women to mix outside the family. Again this is the group in which the father is most likely to bring the child to the consultation. I have even had a male friend of the family bring a child to see me, although he knew nothing about the child or the reason for the consultation, because it was not permitted for the mother to come to the hospital and the father was unable to come. Finally, members of this group usually speak either no English or such poor English that it is difficult to be sure whether they understand what is being said to them. The language difficulty together with the enforced isolation that is inherent in their culture is in my view the main reason why they make poor use of health services.

Even within what might superficially seem to be a fairly uniform group, New York-based male orthodox Jews, Hoffnung found a marked difference between carefully matched tetrads of four sub-sects. These were secular modern orthodox Jews who emphasise secular academic achievement above religious education, traditional modern orthodox Jews for whom secular and religious education are given equal prominence, educated sectarian orthodox Jews whose main education is at a religious seminary, but who attend secular evening classes, and ultra-orthodox Jews whose education is entirely religious with secular education being actively discouraged.[26] In applying two instruments that measure personality and dogmatism, Hoffnung found no significant differences between the first three groups, but he noted that the ultra-orthodox Jews did differ significantly from the other three groups in being 'relatively narrow in interests and stereotyped in thinking; compliant and deferential to authority, custom and tradition; and relatively dogmatic and intolerant'.[26] However, these traits are not inevitably negative. As has been discussed above, Wieselberg found that these very factors assisted in the acceptance and application of her therapy in ultra-orthodox families.[2] Clearly, on the basis of these results, the ultra-orthodox group, with regard for example to its response to disability, is the most likely to 'follow the herd' and react according to the beliefs and practices of the group, rather than take an unpopular line.

Although the results of the above study seem to be clear-cut, Lombroso *et al.* found that in practice this is not so.[27] They studied whether Israeli teenagers would be prepared to work with people with mental illness, have them board in their apartment, or marry them. They found that three main factors defined the groups: place of origin of the family (those from European families being more tolerant than those from families from the Orient), level of education (the better educated being more tolerant than the less well educated) and religious affiliation (the non-religious teenagers being more tolerant than the religious ones). That said, however, although there were significant differences between the groups with regard to willingness to work alongside the mentally ill, as the proposed level of contact became more intimate, the differences in the groups narrowed. Lombroso *et al.* interpret this as meaning that well-educated Western secular Jewish teenagers liked to give an impression of liberality until it actually affected them or their family. However, they comment that those who had actually had personal contact with individuals with mental illness were the most tolerant.[27]

It is implicit in all of the above findings that although religious affiliation, particularly if it is active and devout, affects attitudes to disability or illness in oneself and in others, this is not the only factor involved, and it may not be the main one, since people with and without religious affiliations often have similar attitudes to disability. It may be that local custom, and the knowledge base on which it is founded, are more important. For example, the attitudes of Jews from Middle Eastern backgrounds, where traditional healthcare is more widely used than western medicine, may have more in common with Muslims from the same area than with their co-religionists from Europe.

Although I have stated that people's attitudes to disease and disability are influenced by all aspects of their culture, not just their religion, this obviously plays a major part. In the next chapter I shall consider the teachings of the religions themselves on the question of the cause and management of disability and disease.

References

1 Mundel G (1968) The old beliefs and the cerebral palsied. *Rehabil Record.* **9**(5): 16–21.

2 Wieselberg H (1992) Family therapy and ultra-orthodox Jewish families: a structural approach. *J Fam Therapy.* **14**: 305–29.

3 Strauss RP (1985) Culture, rehabilitation and facial birth defects: international case studies. *Cleft Palate J.* **22**: 56–61.

4 Dein S (1992) Letters to the Rebbe: millennium, messianism and medicine among the Lubavitch of Stamford Hill. *Int J Soc Psychiatry.* **38**: 262–72.

5 Cuninghame CJ, Charlton CPJ and Jenkins SM (1994) Immunisation uptake

and parental perceptions in a strictly orthodox Jewish community in North-east London. *J Pub Health Med.* **16**: 314–17.

6 Law J and Wallfish T (1991) Do minority groups have special needs? Speech therapy and the Chasidic Jewish community in north London. *Child Care Health Dev.* **17**: 319–29.

7 Bilu Y and Witztum E (1994) Culturally sensitive therapy with ultra-orthodox patients: the strategic employment of religious idioms of distress. *Isr J Psychiatry Rel Sci.* **31**: 170–82.

8 Greenberg D and Witztum E (1994) The influence of cultural factors on obsessive-compulsive disorder: religious symptoms in a religious society. *Isr J Psychiatry Rel Sci.* **31**: 211–20.

9 Goshen-Gottstein ER (1987) Mental health implications of living in an ultra-orthodox subculture. *Isr J Psychiatry Rel Sci.* **24**: 145–66.

10 Riddle MA, Scahill L, King R *et al.* (1990) Obsessive-compulsive disorder in children and adolescents: phenomenology and family history. *J Am Acad Child Adolesc Psychiatry.* **29**: 766–72.

11 Swedo SE, Rapoport JL, Leonard H *et al.* (1989) Obsessive-compulsive disorder in children and adolescents: clinical phenomenology in 70 consecutive cases. *Arch Gen Psychiatry.* **46**: 335–41.

12 Akhtar S, Wig NN, Varma VK *et al.* (1975) A phenomenological analysis of symptoms in obsessive-compulsive neurosis. *Br J Psychiatry.* **227**: 342–8.

13 Khanna S and Channabasavanna SM (1988) Phenomenology of obsessions in obsessive-compulsive disorder. *Psychopathology.* **21**: 12–18.

14 Mahgoub OM and Abdel-Hafeiz HB (1991) Pattern of obsessive-compulsive disorder in Eastern Saudi Arabia. *Br J Psychiatry.* **158**: 840–2.

15 Okasha A, Kamel M and Hassan A (1968) Preliminary psychiatric observations in Egypt. *Br J Psychiatry.* **114**: 949–55.

16 Weisner WM and Riffel PA (1960) Scrupulosity: religion and obsessive-compulsive behavior in children. *Am J Psychiatry.* **117**: 314–18.

17 Fallon BA, Liebowitz MR, Hollander E *et al.* (1990) The pharmacotherapy of moral or religious scrupulosity. *J Clin Psychiatry.* **51**: 517–21.

18 Zylbermann R, Landau D and Berson D (1993) The influence of study habits on myopia in Jewish teenagers. *J Paediatr Ophthalmol Strabismus.* **30**: 319–22.

19 Charnes LS and Moore PS (1992) Meeting patients' spiritual needs: the Jewish perspective. *Holistic Nurs Pract.* **6**: 64–72.

20 Zuk GH (1959) The religious factor and the role of guilt in the parental acceptance of the retarded child. *Am J Ment Deficiency.* **64**: 139–47.

21 Zuk GH (1962) The cultural dilemma and spiritual crisis of the family with a handicapped child. *Except Children.* **28**: 405–8.

22 Boles G (1959) Personality factors in mothers of cerebral palsied children. *Genet Psychol Monogr.* **59**: 159–218.

23 Zuk GH, Miller RL, Bartram JB and Kling F (1961) Maternal acceptance of retarded children: a questionnaire study of attitudes and religious background. *Child Dev.* **32**: 525–40.

24 Leyser Y and Dekel G (1991) Perceived stress and adjustment in religious Jewish families with a child who is disabled. *J Psychol.* **125**: 427–38.

25 Watson E (1984) Health of infants and use of health services by mothers of different ethnic groups in East London. *Commun Med.* **6**: 127–35.

26 Hoffnung RA (1975) Personality and dogmatism among selected groups of orthodox Jews. *Psychol Rep.* **37**: 1099–106.

27 Lombroso D, Tyano S and Apter A (1976) Attitudes of the Israeli adolescent to the mentally ill and their treatment. *Isr Ann Psychiatry Rel Disciplines.* **14**: 120–31.

Chapter 4

Religious attitudes to disability

This chapter considers how each of the major western and eastern religions interprets disability in the light of its scriptures and theological traditions.

Young claims that the efficacy of medical practices can be judged on empirical, scientific and symbolic grounds. Empirical proofs are 'confirmed through events in the material world, and explained by coherent sets of ideas'.[1] Contradictions are resolved by invoking special circumstances. For example, the Amhara of Ethiopia explain the failure of an amulet to protect against disease in terms of either a fault in the manufacture of the amulet, or the obliteration of the text in the amulet. This mirrors exactly the explanation given by the Lubavitcher Rebbe for the failure of the Mezuzot on the doorpost to protect the inmates of the house.[2] Young also points out that, in many societies, knowledge is esoteric and is only possessed by 'experts' or magicians.

He defines scientific proof as requiring stringent proof and falsifiable hypotheses, and the results must fit into the broad domain of medical science. He contrasts this with symbolic proof, in which the concern is not so much with how the intervention will affect the sick individual, as with how it will affect all of the people involved in the sickness episode, including relatives and healers. Much illness is self-limiting, so that the intervention of the local healer or shaman is irrelevant, but they are nevertheless credited with the cure. This is not the case only with native healing systems – the dictum of one of my wiser medical teachers was 'beware the fallacy of always attributing the cure to your treatment'. Young also points out that belief in the efficacy of a treatment is not always related to outcome. He cites a study in Taiwan in which 12 patients were observed in treatment by a shaman. Ten of them felt that they were at least partly cured, even though most of them showed no change in symptoms and one was considerably worse. Failure to effect a cure does not necessarily result in loss of belief in the efficacy of the treatment. Often the same treatment affects health and disease, the outcome depending on which is the stronger – the shaman or the causal agent. This is akin to the belief in the Judaeo-Christian religions that if prayer is not followed by cure, God has a different purpose for that person, and His own reason for visiting suffering on him or her.

Young differentiates between *internalising* beliefs, in which the causation of the disease is sought within the patient's body, and *externalising* beliefs, in which the cause is outside the patient. He regards western medicine as a highly organised, internalised belief, seeking physiological explanations, in contrast to the externalised concept that characterises most religious ideas of disease causation and treatment. He cites such pathogenic agencies as grudges that are repaid by witchcraft, but he could equally well have cited a punishment by God for personal or ancestral sin. Because of this type of explanation, the response of the traditional healer will be personal to that episode of sickness and to that person, since the aetiology will be specific and not universal. Thus the aetiology of a heart attack may lie in the failure to spell the word 'heart' correctly in the Mezuzot on that specific person's doorpost, rather than in any more generalisable factor such as diet, smoking history or genetic predisposition.[2]

Traditional Chinese medicine has its own ways of explaining disease and illness. Unschuld defines three explanations for illness (and presumably for disability, too) namely 'causation through other-than-human persons, including gods, demons and ancestors', 'causation through correspondence' (so that, for example, eating a plant that bears no fruit can be contraceptive) and, more familiar to western medicine, 'causation by linear . . . cause-and-effect relationships between natural phenomena'.[3] In our discussion the first and last explanations are relevant, although they are not necessarily mutually exclusive. In defining the cause of the heart attack as a fault in the Mezuzot, the Rebbe did not preclude the use of the full resources of the intensive-care unit to treat it. Zhaojiang, unlike Unschuld, claims that in traditional Confucianism great emphasis is placed on the scientific aspects of traditional Chinese medicine, and reliance on magic and the exorcism of demons for treatment is regarded as unethical.[4] In contrast, McClenon, describing shamanic healing in general, emphasises the power of some individuals (shamans) to use psychic powers to influence external spirits for the harm or benefit of clients, seeing these external forces as causing the disease or affliction.[5]

Up to this point the discussion has concentrated solely on disease and its cure, with the assumption that medicine, whether traditional or western, provides the answer to all health needs. Sevensky differentiates between medicine and healthcare since, he claims, although there is a tendency to medicalise the problems of daily living, 'medicine does not encompass the whole of our efforts to relieve sickness and suffering'.[6] He cites the care of the poor, the old and the handicapped as areas where other aspects of care such as social care, appropriate housing and financial help, are often equally important. He claims a religious basis for this wider type of care, and cites etymological evidence of such words as 'health', 'salvation' and 'holiness' all deriving, in both Greek and Latin, from common roots meaning 'whole'. While acknowledging the historical association between religion and healing institutions, going back as far as the Temples of Asklepios, he sees a deeper basis in the doctrines of the various faiths. For example, in the western Semitic religions, the concept of mankind as part of a creation that is separate from God, and which is therefore not itself sacred and inviolable, allows investigation of mankind himself – that is, it justifies modern scientific and medical enquiry, but with mankind in the role of steward rather than of owner.[4]

Sevensky makes the more contentious claim that all of the world's great religions emphasise the personal freedom to choose.[6] This sits ill with the attitudes of groups such as the Hasidic Jews, who believe that total obedience to the will of God is essential, even if it results in a disastrous situation, for example, an edict that no baby formula could be guaranteed to be kosher, so that if babies could not be breastfed they could not be fed. Far from regarding disability and illness as a distortion of the perfect creation, Sevensky sees it as part of that creation – that the ill or disabled person is as much made in the image of God as is the whole, healthy person, so that this must 'inevitably transform the entire relationship between the two parties [the caregiver and the patient] and make all healthcare a practical recognition of the sanctity of the other'.[6] He points out that in all religions the care of the sick is paramount, and he notes the near-identity of the words of Jesus in the gospel of Matthew, Chapter 25, verse 40, 'in as much as ye have done it unto one of the least of these my brethren, ye have done it unto me' and the teaching of the Buddha, 'whoever . . . would tend me, should tend the sick'.[6]

In contrast, from a conservative Protestant Christian perspective, Mouw views disease as a distortion of the original perfect creation resulting from mankind's sin and rebellion, and that God will rid the creation of it.[7] Despite this, there is also the suggestion that physical suffering is a desirable phenomenon through which God can work (Mouw quotes 2 Corinthians, Chapter 12, verses 7–9, in which Paul rejoices in a thorn in the flesh as a means of demonstrating God's strength through Paul's weakness). He goes further in claiming that 'if medical intervention by experts poses a threat, then it is not to one's autonomy, but rather to one's fidelity to the primary covenantal relationship with God. The danger is not so much a loss of freedom as it is a temptation to place idolatrous trust in medical technology.'[7] Mouw illustrates this by reference to the hypothetical case of a woman with terminal cancer whose doctors think that she should be shielded from the truth of her condition. He argues that if the woman is a Christian she should be told the truth, not because it is her autonomous right, but because it is necessary for her to be able to 'struggle with the spiritual significance of a specific affliction'.[7] The clear implication here is that the causation of the disease is spiritual, and perhaps even that only by confronting this aetiology can this woman be truly healed. By not telling her, the implication is that the doctors are working against her cure.[7]

From some religious viewpoints the question is not whether doctors should tell their patients the truth, for whatever reason, but whether doctors should be involved in the treatment of disease at all. Merrill, speaking from a Christian viewpoint, emphasises the view that illness and disability are the result of sin and rebellion against God. He quotes Ecclesiasticus, Chapter 38, verses 1–6, to support the claim that 'God is the healer and the doctor is his lowly helper'.[8] He claims that so strong was this belief that Pope Gregory the Great discouraged Christian healing because it interfered with God's plan to use sickness as a means of persuading a sinner to repent. He also claims that in the twelfth century the Lateran Council forbade monks to visit the sick or attempt to heal them. Finally, he claims that even 200 years ago, in Catholic countries physicians were forbidden by law to visit a patient who had not confessed his sins to a priest.[8] There seems to be considerable confusion about the role of God in the aetiology of disease and sickness. On the one hand it is claimed that these conditions result from mankind's failure to comply with God's will (i.e. they are man-made), but on the other it is claimed that they are something which God allows as instruments that he can make use of to his own ends. There is also a strong suggestion that medical science is the enemy, and that resorting to it implies lack of faith.

One of the problems faced by those who believe that God uses illness for his own ends is this idea that resorting to medical care may be increasing one's disobedience and thus exacerbating the situation. Hufford has examined the concept of illness as a response by God to sin, and the use made by God of suffering, against the background of theodicy (if God is good and all powerful, why do the innocent suffer?).[9] He attempts to show that, given the original premises that scripture is true and that miraculous healing occurs, two pathways follow, 'you will be healed' and 'you may be healed'.[9] In the first pathway, healing is certain if by your own action you can remove the cause of the illness, the result of personal sin and therefore not innocent. Only by expiating the sin by faith and correct prayer can the cause be removed. If your faith is sufficient to do this, you *will* be healed. Reliance on medical care indicates weak faith. If you are not healed, you have not expiated the sin. This can have a damaging effect, even on those who do not themselves believe it. For example, when physiotherapy was offered to physically disabled children in the care of Mother Teresa's nuns in Calcutta, it was refused on the grounds that the love of God was sufficient for their needs and made physiotherapy irrelevant.[10] In the second pathway, suffering is regarded as the result of mankind's imperfection rather than of personal sin. If you do pray for healing, God may choose to heal miraculously, or may use medical care as his instrument. Either way, you *may* be healed. To use medical care therefore shows no lack of faith.

It is often implied that religious belief, and in particular the way in which that belief affects the believer's attitude to such things as causation and treatment of illness and disability, is a minority concern and is something which need not impinge on general attitudes to such matters. Harakas argues that the religious dimension in bioethics is no more idiosyncratic than the secular dimension, and that to take religious views into account when discussing ethical issues in medicine is no more a minority attempting to force its opinions on the majority than it is if secular views are taken into account.[11] Furthermore, although there is diversity among the different religions, this is not as great as it seems, since most if not all religions start from the assumption that there is a transcendent being from whom morality flows, and who supersedes human opinion. Harakas emphasises that throughout orthodox Christian theology there is the theme of community. The Godhead itself is a community of Father, Son and Holy Spirit. If Man is made in the image of God, and is fulfilled in imitation of God, then 'since God is a community of persons, human life can only find its fulfilment in a communal and community existence'.[11] Unlike Mouw's conception, where the reliance on divine intervention in the healing process may set up barriers between church and medicine, Harakas claims that the whole concept of the hospital originated in the Eastern Orthodox church, the monks employing secular physicians to provide free medical care for the poor, priest physicians serving equally at altar and sick bed, and the physician saints, the Holy Unmercenaries, giving their expertise free to the poor. He sees the doctrine of original sin and the fallenness of mankind not as the result of individual or ancestral guilt, but as 'aspects of our human condition which are broken, distorted, corrupt and self-deceptive'.[11] It is therefore not the source of disease and disability, but something which should 'equip the ethicist with a certain cautious suspicion'.[11]

Keown and Keown take this theme of the religious life as a community further by attempting to demonstrate that all of the world's major religions share a common ethic by comparing the Buddhist and Christian attitudes to euthanasia.[12] Since both religions regard life as sacred, they claim that both religions forbid any action or omission which is specifically designed to end a human life, whatever apparent benefit accrues to the patient. To support this, they quote the Epistle to the Romans, Chapter 3, verses 7 and 8, in which Paul denies that one can do evil that good may result, and the Buddhist Monastic Rule on taking human life promulgated to counteract suicides and requests to be killed by others among monks disgusted by their bodies. This expressly forbids both the killing of a human being and seeking help in dying. This is extended in a fifth-century commentary by Buddhaghosa to cover the issue of quality of life in two situations, terminal illness and long-term disability. According to Buddhaghosa, even suggesting to a dying monk that death would be preferable to his present condition was wrong in that the monks who did this had made death their aim. Keown and Keown make the point that this does not mean in either tradition that life must be preserved at all costs and by all means, even if the means are futile or unreasonably burdensome.[12]

Perrett questioned the accuracy of some of these statements and takes issue with Keown and Keown on the basis that they do not clearly define what they mean by Buddhism, euthanasia and the sanctity of life.[13] He also claims that the Keowns are factually incorrect in claiming that to kill or to seek death results in lifelong excommunication. He states that the ordinances that they use apply only to monks, and that the lifelong exclusion is from the monastic order only, not from lay Buddhism.

It is instructive to compare the two definitions of euthanasia. For Perrett it is 'the killing of those who are incurably ill and in great pain or distress, where the killing is done for the sake of those killed, and in order to spare them further suffering or distress',[13] whereas for Keown and Keown it is 'the intentional killing of a patient by act or omission as part of his or her medical care. We are not concerned therefore with the administration of palliative drugs, or the withdrawal of futile or excessively burdensome treatment which may, as a foreseen side-effect, hasten death'.[12] For both, therefore, the sanctity of life is not absolute, to be preserved at all costs, and the motive plays a morally relevant part. However, although for both the motive is all-important, for Perrett it is justifiable to kill deliberately in order to relieve suffering, whereas for the Keowns the primary motive is not to cause death but to relieve suffering, death being a secondary result of the action taken – the so-called *doctrine of double effect*. Boyle, a Roman Catholic, uses the doctrine of double effect to claim that some moral standpoints, such as that of the natural law philosophy of the Catholic church, result in radical moral disagreement which cannot be resolved, since some things, for example, the stand against abortion or euthanasia, or against homosexuality, are absolute and so cannot be compromised.[14] This is again based on the Epistle to the Romans, Chapter 3, verse 8. Perrett points out that voluntary euthanasia at least, that is, euthanasia at the specific request of the sufferer, is akin to assisted suicide, and that Buddhism in general is less antagonistic to suicide than is Christianity. Suicide out of despair is seen as prudential, in that the suicide will be reborn with the original karma unresolved, and suicide by a monk that is well motivated, such as the self-immolation of Thich Quang Duc in Saigon,[15] is a praiseworthy act. More recently, the Dalai Lama has decreed that if the prolongation of a life is *only* going to cause difficulties and suffering for others, by which he presumably means that it will have no other effect, it may be terminated, and Kalu Rinpoche has decreed that it is a karmically neutral act for a terminally ill patient to take himself or be taken off a life-support system (both references are quoted by Perrett[13]). This is a surprising judgement, since presumably it also leaves unresolved karma. On the question of whether Buddhism regards all lives as equally valuable, Perrett also quotes Bhuddaghosa, who states that 'in the case of humans, the killing is more blameworthy the more virtuous they are'.[13]

Where does this leave the Buddhist attitude to the disabled person? Since our present life is determined by our karma, the balance of good and evil deeds performed in past incarnations, then it must be that disability, as part of the whole of life, is the direct result of past and present sin. This is a doctrine that is also common to Hinduism. In a paper discussing the interaction of karma and theodicy, Sharma claims that karma gives a coherent answer – that suffering is the just reward for past misdeeds, committed in past lives and unresolved.[16] However, although suffering is in a sense the fault of the sufferer, and should therefore result in both suffering and guilt, this is often not the case because deeds committed in a past life are unknowable, and therefore the present incarnation cannot be held responsible for them. This weakens Sharma's claim to coherence, since she seems to be claiming that disability is the fault of the disabled, but simultaneously that it is a fault for which they cannot be held responsible.[16]

To talk of the Jewish attitude to disability could be seen as misleading in that it could imply that Judaism is a unified entity in which all who claim to be Jewish will have the same conception of disability. In most forms of Judaism, from the non-practising secular Jew, through liberal, reformed and conservative Judaism to orthodox Judaism, secular education runs alongside religious education and is seen to be at least as important as the latter. There are, in the main, no objections to these children attending secular schools, or Jewish schools maintained by the secular authority, or attending appropriate clinics. Even among the orthodox Jews, although marrying out of the Jewish community is frowned upon, marriages are not usually arranged, and there is not the imperative to hide a disabled member of the family. However, for the ultra-orthodox Jews, the haredim, problems do arise.

The main difference between the other groups and the haredim lies in the weight placed on the Law, Halacha. For liberal, reformed and conservative Jews this is one of the pillars (not necessarily the most important one) that regulates how life should be lived. However, for orthodox and haredic Jews it is the primary guide, although there is a difference in emphasis. Whereas both groups hold that 'orthodoxy involves belief . . . that the Five Books of Moses are the unmediated [i.e. directly dictated] word of God',[17] they would disagree on how this is applied to daily life. An orthodox Jew 'will consult a rabbi if he has a question regarding a point of halacha, and will be bound by the rabbi's ruling. He might consult with a rabbi on a problem unrelated to halacha, but that would be by way of seeking advice; there would be no binding authority in the rabbi's response. A haredi, on the other hand, will consult his rabbi or Hasidic Rebbe on every aspect of his life, and will obey the advice he receives as though it were an halachic ruling.'

The other characteristic of haredism is the emphasis placed on the study of the Talmud. This is undertaken not just as a means of understanding the religion, but as an end in itself. It is not only a mitzvah – it is the greatest mitzvah.[17] Fulfilling this mitzvah is incumbent on all haredi, not just on rabbis or Halakhic lawyers. It is this that creates one of the greatest difficulties in providing adequate special educational or health provision to disabled children within this community. In order to fulfil the needs for Talmudic study, the children attend a multiplicity of sectarian religious schools, where such provision is difficult. Therefore when trying to understand how disability is seen from their viewpoint, it is necessary to take into account the fact that, for the Haredim, all aspects of life are tightly governed by total obedience to the Law as interpreted in the Talmud.

In general, the Jewish attitude to impairment, disability and handicap is complex. On the one hand, all life is regarded as infinitely precious, having been made in the image of God,[18] and since infinity is indivisible, no one life is any more or less valuable than any other, regardless of its quality. On the other hand, it is part of the Law that those with a blemish, such as the blind, lame or deformed, should be excluded from offering the bread in the temple (Leviticus, Chapter 21, verses 17–20), which implies that there is a gradation in worth. That there is such a gradation is emphasised in attitudes to treatment. In a paper defining Jewish attitudes to mental illness, Aviner points out the fundamental difference between the psychiatrist, whose desire is to establish the diagnosis and treatment as soon as possible in order to prevent deterioration, and the Talmudist, who is concerned to decide whether the disabled person is fit to remain a part of the community, with legal and religious responsibilities, even though to remove him may hasten that individual's collapse.[19] This implies that not only may some disabled people be incapable of exercising ritual duties, but also they may not even be fit to remain a part of the community in general. Greenberg and Witztum have pointed out that in the ultra-orthodox communities, responsa from several rabbis explicitly state that the advice tendered by psychiatrists and psychologists in the treatment of mental illness offends the Torah.[20] The responsa also contain evidence of the beliefs about aetiology. For instance, 'Even the best therapists have nothing to offer those whose sins have brought them to depression or sadness, for the help they need is from those knowledgeable in Tora, who are the real healers of souls'.[20] However, not all illness is considered to be of this form. Levin claims that although there is good biblical evidence for the idea that illness results from sin and is the divine punishment for sin, earthly causes are also given, notably contagion or possession by spirits.[21] He further claims that the Talmud rejects the idea that illness is a visitation from God as a result of sin and that in the Talmud 'physicians were forbidden to increase a patient's distress by saying that his illness was a consequence of his sins'.[21]

Different religious conceptions of the nature and cause of illness inevitably lead to different attitudes to treatment. Zohar discusses the difference in opinion between two medieval rabbis.[22] Maimonides maintained that the practice of medicine was legitimate, as part of God's will, whereas Nahmanides held that it was an interference with God's will, and was only necessary at all because of lack of faith on the part of the patient. The followers of Nahmanides, Zohar claims, take the injunction in Exodus, Chapter 21, verse 19, that an assailant 'must . . . pay for his victim's healing: and he shall cause him to be thoroughly healed', as permission to heal but not to be healed. The argument seems to be that because people have become used to being healed by physicians rather than turning to God in order to find the cause of and remedy for their suffering, it is permitted for physicians to heal them.[22]

Furthermore, Zohar cites a modern interpretation of a thirteenth-century sage, Bahye ben Asher, that permission to heal does not extend to internal medicine, since this is assumed to be independent of man's intervention and therefore solely caused by divine intervention. This has interesting implications for disability. The claim is that only man-made conditions, such as a wound or injury, may be treated by physicians. This can be extended to those diseases caused by disordered lifestyle. 'If this is granted, then the class of God-induced ailments consists of only a congenital illness . . . or from the weakness and dysfunction of particular organs.'[22] Clearly, since most of the impairments that cause disability fall within this class, the implication is that divine permission for physicians to heal does not extend to the causes of disability. Yet even this is not clear-cut. A 'second restriction . . . is that any illness whose nature and cure are clear is not considered an internal illness induced by heaven'.[22] This presumably means that the term 'internal' can be used as a synonym for 'not understood', so that as we learn more of the mechanism of disabling conditions they begin to fall within the class of conditions that even the followers of Nahmanides would allow to be treated.

Jewish attitudes to disabled people pervade not only assessment of the fitness of such people to remain members of the community, but also the behaviour of those deemed to be so fit in relation to the rest of the community, and the community's behaviour towards them. Jakobovits enlarges on the duty of a Jew to ensure that his or her potential marriage partner is healthy.[23] Among the attributes to be looked for in the future spouse and their family are the absence of even a hidden blemish, such that the wife-to-be is required to submit to an examination in the bathhouse by the prospective husband's female relatives. There is also an injunction not to marry the daughter of an ignoramus. Jakobovits supports the latter injunction by reference to Deuteronomy, Chapter 27, verse 21: 'Cursed be he who lieth with any manner of beast'.[23] The clear implication is that the mentally retarded are to be regarded as beasts. In the same chapter it is stated that according to the Talmud it is not lawful to marry into a family in which there have been at least three epileptics or lepers. Rashi is said to have extended this to any hereditary disease. Since in Jakobovits' text the word 'hereditary' is in parentheses, it may be that the original extended the prohibition to any disease. 'Insane persons' cannot contract valid marriages at all, nor can 'lunatics', although apparently on the grounds that such a marriage could not be happy or peaceful, rather than for eugenic reasons.[23]

Other attitudes to disability can be found in concessions allowed to the sick. Thus, for instance, the blind are not allowed to carry a stick on the Sabbath if it is not indispensable to walking but *only acts as a guide* (my italics). An orthodox Jewish optometrist recently told me that he advises his patients not to wear contact lenses on the Sabbath, since if they fell out it would be against the Law to pick them up.

On the other hand, we have seen the strand in Jewish thought that emphasises the equal worth of all people. Newman discusses the unique position of human life, given that God created man in his image (Genesis, Chapter 1, verse 27).[24] Because of this, Newman argues, human life is uniquely sacred, which generates three major principles – it possesses intrinsic and infinite value, the preservation of life is the highest moral imperative, and all lives are equal. All arguments based on quality of life are invalid. Since all human lives are equal, selecting one individual against another to receive or be denied a scarce resource is never justified, and only a random allocation among people of equal need can be justified.[24] However, Golding disputes this and suggests that, for example, in attempting to decide which of two patients who need the sole respirator or kidney machine available should get it, a hierarchy of priority could be drawn up: 'A youth before an old man, a healthy old man before a sick person, a sick person before a mortally ill person, and the latter before someone who is moribund'.[25] This dilemma – that all lives are equal in the sight of God, but that hierarchies of worth exist – is one that cannot easily be resolved, and it is certainly not settled in traditional or indeed even in modern Jewish writings.[25]

Investigation of the cause of disability also causes problems, since all forms of genetic testing, even a simple karyotype, can cause difficulty for some Hasidic families, as they are likely to lead to genetic counselling and thus the temptation to limit fertility. However, they do support premarital screening. Jakobovits makes the point that preventing the marriage of two people who are likely to conceive a disabled child ensures that the marriage partner is healthy, and is qualitatively different from genetic advice aimed at limiting the fertility of an already married couple.[23]

One of the main concerns of this book, namely the criteria for the allocation of scarce resources, is – as Newman points out – hardly touched upon in modern Jewish writings. He attributes this to the fact that the Jewish legal tradition is not meant to apply to non-Jews, and since Jews have never been in a position of overall authority over non-Jews, the possibility of requiring them to conform to Jewish law has never arisen.[24] This situation is changing to some extent in Israel, where the religious parties are politically strong and non-Jewish citizens are required to adhere to Jewish law. Furthermore, it is not acceptable to choose one individual to receive a resource over another, since all are equal, and therefore equally entitled, in the sight of God. As we saw, one view would be that where equality was impossible, anything but random allocation of resources would imply a discrimination between people on the grounds of worth.

Therefore although it is claimed that all life – healthy or not – is equal in the sight of God, and must thus be so in the sight of man, there are in fact many strictures placed on those who are disabled. These range from the direct, such as the ban on holding ritual office, to the indirect, which result, for example, from the rules about marrying into the family of a disabled person, which can have a major influence on the general attitude to disability. The emphasis that is placed on the need for all aspects of life, including treatment of the disabled person, to conform to the dictates of the Law, may not only cause conflict about the site of such treatment, for example, whether in a secular or religious school, but may also restrict access to the treatment, if the method, for example, psychoanalysis, is regarded as inimical to the religion.

Within most strictly observed religions, not just Judaism, there is an element of compulsion to comply with the dictates of the deity, and this is particularly so in observant Judaism, and paramount in Hasidism. This not only influences the perceived causality of suffering, but also determines what is acceptable treatment, which may result in the members of the religion demanding a disproportionate amount of the available resources, not strictly because of the needs of the treatment, but because of the need for the treatment to be conducted in a specific way. Consequently, the physician may be placed in the difficult position of having his or her treatment plan dictated by non-clinical considerations.

It is difficult to find any comment on Islam and disability. Rispler-Chaim, writing on Islamic medical ethics, comments that this has never been an independent field of study within Islam.[26] The only reference to disability in that author's paper is an oblique one, namely that in response to an attempt by the Egyptian government to impose birth control, a fatwa was issued that this could only be justified in highly fertile women or women with genetic or mental disease. No mention is made of women who have given birth to disabled children.[26]

On a more general level, everything that happens (good or bad) is under the control of God. As Haneef says, 'In human life, ease and suffering alike, and the events which produce them, equally have a purpose and meaning, and are equally a part of God's infinitely wise plan for His creation. . . . God alone is the source of benefit or harm, and turning to anyone . . . other than Him for help . . . is not only futile, but . . . attributes to others powers which God alone possesses.'[27] This would seem to imply a fatalistic approach to handicap and disability, which God will alleviate or not according to his will, but Haneef denies that this is so on the grounds that since man does not know his fate, he must do his best to help himself. Whether this implies that he can seek medical care is unclear. Distress and trouble borne patiently are viewed as expiation for sin, leading to reward in the hereafter.

In all of the religions discussed above it is clear that disability and suffering imply to some extent blame on someone's part – either the person who is suffering, the community in general, which has collectively transgressed, or the ancestors or previous incarnations of the sufferer. Attached to blame is guilt, so that management of disability within a religious community will often imply that the suffering is deserved and perhaps should therefore be borne. On the other hand, compassion is also a part of the teachings of all of the major religions, and such activities as caring for the sick, giving alms to the poor and generally helping those less fortunate than oneself are all regarded as praiseworthy religious activities, or even as religious duties.

In general, therefore, there is no conflict between the religious and secular authorities with regard to the need to care for disabled children, and to ensure that they receive the facilities they need in order to overcome their disability as far as is possible.

References

1 Young A (1980) An anthropological perspective on medical knowledge. *J Med Phil.* **5**: 102–16.

2 Dein S (1992) Letters to the Rebbe: millennium, messianism and medicine among the Lubavitch of Stamford Hill. *Int J Soc Psychiatry.* **38**: 262–72.

3 Unschuld PU (1980) Concepts of illness in ancient China: the case of demonological medicine. *J Med Phil.* **5**: 117–31.

4 Zhaojiang G (1995) Chinese Confucian culture and the medical ethical tradition. *J Med Ethics.* **21**: 239–46.

5 McClenon J (1993) The experiential foundations of Shamanic healing. *J Phil Med.* **18**: 107–27.

6 Sevensky RI (1983) The religious foundations of health care: a conceptual approach. *J Med Ethics.* **9**: 165–9.

7 Mouw RJ (1979) Biblical revelation and medical decisions. *J Med Phil.* **4**: 367–82.

8 Merrill GG (1981) Health, healing and religion. *MD State Med J.* **30**(12): 45–7.

9 Hufford DJ (1993) Epistemologies in religious healing. *J Med Phil.* **18**: 175–94.

10 Roberts J (1999) *Abdul's Taxi to Kalighat.* Profile Books, London.

11 Harakas SS (1993) An Eastern Orthodox approach to bioethics. *J Med Phil.* **18**: 531–48.

12 Keown D and Keown J (1995) Killing, karma and caring: euthanasia in Buddhism and Christianity. *J Med Ethics.* **21**: 265–9.

13 Perrett RW (1996) Buddhism, euthanasia and the sanctity of life. *J Med Ethics.* **22**: 309–13.

14 Boyle J (1994) Radical moral disagreement in contemporary health care. *J Med Phil.* **19**: 183–200.

15 Hanh TN (1967) *Vietnam: the lotus in the sea of fire.* SCM Press Ltd, London.

16 Sharma U (1978) Theodicy and the doctrine of karma. In: W Foy (ed.) *Man's Religious Quest.* Croom Helm, London, p. 33.

17 Landau D (1993) *Piety and Power: the world of Jewish fundamentalism.* Secker & Warburg, London.

18 Jakobovits I (1986) The Jewish contribution to medical ethics. In: P Byrne (ed.) *Rights and Wrongs in Medicine.* King's Fund, London, pp. 115–26.

19 Aviner S (1990) Stigmatisation in traditional Jewish sources. *Med Law.* **9**: 1246–9.

20 Greenberg D and Witztum E (1994) Ultra-orthodox Jewish attitudes towards mental health care (editorial). *Isr J Psychiatry Rel Sci.* **31**: 143–4.

21 Levin S (1973) Jewish ethics in relation to medicine. *S Afr Med J.* **47**: 924–30.

22 Zohar NJ (1995) Human action and God's will: a problem of consistency in Jewish bio-ethics. *J Med Phil.* **20**: 387–402.

23 Jakobovits I (1975) *Jewish Medical Ethics.* Bloch, New York, pp. 155, 156.

24 Newman LE (1992) Jewish theology and bioethics. *J Med Phil.* **17**: 309–27.

25 Golding MP (1983) Preventive vs. curative medicine: perspectives of the Jewish legal tradition. *J Med Phil.* **8**: 269–86.

26 Rispler-Chaim V (1989) Islamic medical ethics in the twentieth century. *J Med Ethics.* **15**: 203–8.

27 Haneef S (1979) *What Everyone Should Know About Islam and Muslims.* Kazi Publications, Lahore.

Chapter 5

The concept of harm

Providing for disabled children in communities such as the Hasidim while as far as possible respecting the religious requirements of the community raises three questions. First, is harm done to the child if religious beliefs prevent optimum treatment? Secondly, is harm done to the child if religious beliefs are bypassed in the management of his or her disability? Thirdly, if harm is done to the child because of the religious beliefs, is this harm greater for a disabled child than for an able-bodied child?

Although a dictionary definition of 'harm' as damage or hurt, and thus of 'harmful' as something which causes damage or hurt,[1] provides a starting point, it is necessary to relate the idea of harm to the effect that it has on individuals. Can impeding what is beneficial be said to be harmful? Can depriving a person of potential benefit, even if doing so does not alter the status quo, be harmful? Feinberg defines harm as the invasion of a person's interest, and since most people have an interest in not being hurt or offended, he would claim that hurt or offence is always harmful, although harm is not always hurtful or offensive.[2] If you have no knowledge of the invasion and therefore are not hurt or offended by it, you are nevertheless harmed. Feinberg uses two examples to illustrate this. The first is that the fact that you do not know you have been burgled, because you are away on holiday, does not mean that you have not been harmed by the burglar. This is similar to an example in which I used the case of a crook falsely and successfully claiming an inheritance of which the rightful heir was unaware to argue that even if one is unaware of a benefit, being deprived of it is harmful. Harm is done and the interests of the rightful heir are invaded.[3] The second of Feinberg's examples supports the idea that what you do not know cannot hurt you, but it can harm you. If a man is being cuckolded by his wife, he will not be hurt by this if he knows nothing about it. It is the knowledge itself that is hurtful. However, he is being harmed in that his interest in a stable relationship with his wife is being invaded.

Not all authorities accept such a broad definition of harm as to include invasion of any interest and would restrict it to actual physical or mental injury,[4] but in my view this is too restrictive.

Can the State use coercion to prevent harm? Feinberg claims that since coercion can be seen as a 'harm-causing evil', then it can only be justified if 'it is necessary for the prevention of even greater evils'.[2] He calls this the 'harm to others principle (. . . harm principle) which permits society to restrict the liberty of some persons in order to prevent harm to others'. If it is permissible to use coercion to prevent one citizen from harming another, is it also permissible to use coercion to compel one citizen to benefit another, for example, taxing one person in order to provide education for another, and is failure to do this the commission of a harm? If one holds that 'being without something good is a mere non-benefit, whereas being in possession of something evil is a harm',[2] then not receiving an education can be seen as a non-benefit rather than as a harm. However, if you are deprived of all food you are just as harmed, you die, as if you were fed poisoned food. From this Feinberg concludes that 'Harm . . . can consist in a lack as well as a presence . . . an omission as well as an action'.[2] Must the thing of which one is deprived be a need, or can it be merely a desire? A millionaire cannot be said to need the few pounds lost in petty larceny, but he is harmed by it. Feinberg therefore defines the harm principle in such a way that 'changes in the condition of a protectable interest in harmful directions count as a kind of harm, the prevention of which . . . may justify coercion. However, when harms have to be ranked . . . an actual injurious condition should outweigh a mere change in a harmful direction'.[2]

The fact that harm can accrue from unmet needs inevitably raises the question of what constitutes a need. Does the demonstration of a need always imply that failure to meet it causes harm, and if not, under what circumstances does it do so? There is an intuitive sense of rightness in the claim that, in a society in which resources are limited, need will confer rights and will be the overriding criterion by which such resources as there are will be distributed. However, there are certain assumptions underlying this statement – that needs can be defined in a way which brooks no disagreement, or that it is essential that needs are met.

What then constitutes a need? In common parlance, the word has varying force. 'I need a breath of fresh air' does not have the urgency of 'I need oxygen to live'. Again it is necessary to differentiate between needs and desires. The word 'need' as used in 'I need a swimming pool in my back garden' could be changed to 'want' or 'desire' without changing the meaning, unless it could be demonstrated that a swimming pool was necessary as a means of therapy for cerebral palsy, for example. On the other hand, to make such a substitution in 'I need food to survive' would be nonsense. However, as Daniels points out, 'we refer to the means of reaching any of our goals as needs'.[5] If a need is anything required to achieve a goal, then the differentiation should perhaps not be between need and desire, but between the relative importance of the goal. Although there appears to be an obvious difference in the above two examples of a need for a pool, both of them actually have a goal – the first to enable me to compete with the neighbours, and the second to enable me to improve my state of health. The difference lies in the relative importance of the goals. Wiggins and Derman claim that it is not 'needs being less "subjective" than mere desire, but to the role of need in bringing out what is vital to human beings in questions of the distribution of benefits and burdens'.[6]

This raises a second difficulty, namely who makes the decision as to what constitutes a goal that is sufficiently important to result in a need which must be met. Is it the person who is providing for the need, the person with the need, or some other agency: society, the Government, the paymaster? Daniels suggests that for a need to confer a right, objective criteria which invoke 'a measure of importance independent of the individual's own assessment'[5] should be applied.

Willard disputes the assumption that a need is a discoverable fact about a person rather than a value judgement.[7] He points out that needs are often a means to an end, and since a means is a discoverable fact, needs are also regarded as facts. He uses a tooth filling as an example: 'If I say I need a filling in my tooth, it is the filling, not my need, which is a means to a desirable goal – less pain, healthy teeth, etc. The cavity in my tooth is a fact about me, and the filling is, or will be, a fact about me. But there is not another fact about me called a need I have for a filling.'[7] He also takes issue with Fletcher's definition that 'rights are nothing but formal recognition by society of certain human needs'[7] on the grounds that both are values, neither are facts, and each must be balanced against the other. This is particularly pertinent as it is precisely because the values of some religious groups differ from those of the host community that difficulties in defining needs arise. Willard points out that advances such as bypass surgery start as a luxury, and then come to be seen as a necessity, and therefore as a need. He claims that if such needs are truly facts, then they would have been as much a need for a caveman as for a modern executive. Although today we can say that some cavemen would have benefited from bypass surgery, they could not have had a need for something that did not then exist. Willard claims that this concept of health need can lead to a thing being done because it can be. Thus, for example, the existence of the means of prolonging life in a given patient means that he has a need for them, even if prolonging his life has no meaning for him, or indeed may cause him additional suffering.

Acheson defines two approaches to the fulfilment of need, namely the humanitarian and the realistic approach.[8] He introduces the concept of the service equivalent of need, which can be used to meet that need, for example, a consultation, medicine, or the use of an ambulance or a hospital bed. The humanitarian approach identifies human suffering as a need that must be alleviated, defines the service equivalent that is required, and then seeks the resources necessary to provide it. If this was applied to groups like the Hasidim, then the fact that they identified a need would imply that the resources required must be found to meet it. The realistic approach defines the resources available; this defines what service equivalents can be provided, and thus what needs can be sought. According to this model there is little point in surveying a developing country for the incidence of varicose veins if there are no resource equivalents to provide the treatment that is needed. The weakness of this argument is that the resources are themselves defined by a hierarchy of need, and it may be that the powers that be have determined that armaments or bolstering the president's private bank balance are greater needs. On the other hand, surveys of the need for artificial hips in the UK can be justified because the discovered need can be met with the resources available. According to this model the patient only has the right to what can be provided. As a corollary of this, if no effective remedy for the need is available, then there is no requirement for the need to be met. This would, for example, cover the caveman and heart bypass example, since as this treatment was not available at that time there was no duty to provide it.

A further problem is that of defining whose is the need. Moore uses triage as an example of distribution according to need, a technique that was developed in medicine by the military.[9] He implies that this allows individuals with the greatest need to receive priority treatment. This is of course the reverse of what actually happens on the battlefield, since the need there is to return as many men as possible to the firing line as quickly as possible. Priority is therefore given to the lightly wounded who can be patched up to fight again, followed by those who can be given minimal treatment and sent back to hospitals behind the lines, by which time the dying are dead and require no resources. The need here is clearly that of the restricted society of the battlefield, to which the need of the individual is totally subservient. In general, however, the well-being of individuals is usually directly linked to the well-being of society – precisely the claim that would be made by the Hasidic community to justify the perceived need for their children to be educated in their own schools.

One of the central problems is to define the conflict of need between the religious communities and the wider community. From the view-point of the latter, when deciding what services should be provided to a disabled child, the need is to make a detailed assessment of the child, to perform whatever investigations are necessary in order to make a diagnosis, and then to define a programme of management and treatment in association with the local education and health authorities. From the viewpoint of the Hasidic family, the need is to do all that is necessary which does not conflict with the Law of God. Thus, for example, investigations are resisted on the grounds that they may result in a genetic diagnosis which will lead to the offer of genetic counselling, and then of prenatal diagnosis and induced abortion, or other forms of fertility limitation, which are forbidden. Similarly, attendance at a secular school interferes with the religious element of education, so that any management which is to be conducted in school has to be within the private Jewish system, even if it is provided by the state health and education services. Difficulties arise even in management that is conducted in local assessment centres. Many families refuse to attend these centres because it draws attention to the presence of disability in the family, and so prejudices the marriageability of other members of the family. Even those who do attend have difficulties. For example, group physiotherapy may not be acceptable for a mixed-sex group over the age of three years, since it usually involves removing the outer clothing.

Daniels, quoting Braybrooke, differentiates between 'course-of-life needs' which people have 'all through their lives or at certain stages of life through which all must pass', such as food, shelter, etc., and 'adventitious needs' which are 'things we need because of the particular contingent projects . . . on which we embark', deficiency of the former 'endangering the normal functioning of the subject . . . considered as a member of a natural species'.[5] Braybrooke takes a very biological view of course-of-life needs. If lack of a particular resource brings the course-of-life to an end, it is a course-of-life need. Thus food and oxygen are course-of-life needs, whereas education is not. The dilemma then is this. For the Hasidic community, to adhere to the Law of God is the paramount course-of-life need, which must be met above all others if the child is to function as a normal human being. Yet for the wider community it is no more than an adventitious need, which puts no obligation on the health and education authorities. To define cultural and religious factors as course-of-life needs extends Braybrooke's idea. It can be extended even further. If a course-of-life need is not met then this causes course-of-life harm. However, failure to meet an adventitious need causes only adventitious harm. Therefore the nub of the problem is reaching a compromise on how the different parties define 'course-of-life' and 'adventitious'.

Two factors are pertinent here. First, under British law, if the educational needs of a child cannot be met by the ordinary resources of a mainstream school, then a Statement of Educational Need must be made which defines what the child's needs are and where they are to be met.[10] Since most education authorities maintain religious schools, religion is presumably regarded as an educational need. Secondly, the World Health Organization definition of handicap is 'a disadvantage . . . that prevents the fulfilment of a role that is normal (depending on age, sex, and social and *cultural factors*) for that individual' (my italics).[11] Therefore for the education and health authorities the perceived needs of this community can only be met by diverting resources, to the detriment of others. A secondary problem for the authorities is that none of the private Jewish schools have been approved by the Department of Education and Science, partly because they are often staffed by unqualified teachers, and partly because the type of education that is offered usually precludes the acquisition of statutory leaving examinations, so further education other than within the Hasidic tradition is impossible. The question here is whether accepting the parents' definition of the needs of the child is in fact in the best interest of the child, or whether it in fact causes him or her harm. Furthermore, in attempting to exercise the right to special educational provision on their own terms, it could perhaps be claimed that there is then a corresponding duty on the Hasidic community to minimise this harm by ensuring that their schools do meet the standards required of secular schools.

The second of the original assumptions was that needs confer rights and therefore must necessarily be met. Is this so? If one person has a need, does this necessarily imply that someone else has a corresponding obligation to meet that need? Here again the distinction between course-of-life needs and adventitious needs is helpful. Some course-of-life needs are universally applicable (e.g. food and oxygen), since their lack brings the course-of-life to an end. If the word 'community' means anything at all, then there is an obligation for these needs to be met by the community. In addition to these life-sustaining universal course-of-life needs, I would suggest that the idea can be extended by allowing the community to define other course-of-life needs (e.g. access to adequate housing, clothing, education, etc.). In so doing they will take on the obligation to meet these needs, either altruistically or through the application of the law, such as the 1981 Education Act, thereby in effect conferring a right. The Hasidic Jews have acted in this way by defining obedience to the Law of God not only as a course-of-life need, but also for them as the primary course-of-life need from which all others flow. This was dramatically demonstrated some years ago when it was decided by one of the smaller groups that no baby formula could be guaranteed to be kosher, since none could be guaranteed to be completely free of animal flesh. It was therefore decreed that no formula could be fed to babies within that group, even though this meant that some babies could not be fed at all. To keep the Law was paramount, whereas keeping the babies alive was in the hands of God, who provided the means of doing both through one of the local (non-Jewish) paediatricians, who established a bank of wet nurses! Even within the Hasidic tradition a case could be made that the group was acting unlawfully, since they were putting the babies' lives at risk, and even the Law of God can be broken in order to save a life. However, the obligation to obey the Law is paramount only for Jews, because of the unique relationship between them and God.[12] Gentiles are neither required nor expected to obey the Law. The course-of-life need is defined by the Jewish community and applies only to them. It therefore extends the concept further by making a course-of-life need selective rather than universal.

The proposition is that lack of treatment and alienation from one's family and culture do cause harm, and that conversely, receiving treatment and belonging to a family are benefits. I shall produce no empirical evidence that this is so, nor shall I produce evidence that therapy can be effective. The first point is central to the religious position, and neither side disputes the second point. If, as Sacks argues, the family and especially the religiously based family is the fundamental unit of society, and to break this down causes immeasurable harm both to the individual and to society,[13] then anything which militates against such belonging – even the management of disability – has the potential, at least, for harm. On the other hand, if it is accepted that giving therapy and treatment to a disabled child is beneficial in that it will enable the development of skills that would otherwise be impossible, then anything which militates against such provision is also potentially harmful.

The concept of harm may be culturally and geographically dependent – what is considered to be harmful in one culture or locality will not necessarily be considered to be so in another. For example, while on holiday in Turkey, a 13-year-old English girl met and married a 16-year-old Turkish boy, in a religious (but not civil) ceremony, with her parents' blessing. Her local Social Services department in England made her a Ward of Court, and demanded that she return to the UK and the marriage be declared invalid, on the grounds that it was illegal in British and Turkish law for a 13-year-old to marry or have sexual intercourse. The girl's response was that she had chosen to live in Turkey, where she was made to feel beautiful and loved, rather than rejected and unloved as she felt in England. Within the community in which she was living, such marriages are so commonplace and well regarded that, although they are technically illegal, no action is ever taken by the authorities to prevent them. The response to the alleged harm caused by this marriage is therefore threefold. In the UK, the girl is regarded as a child, unable to enter into the marriage contract and needing to be protected against sexual abuse. The harm is seen as so great that it justifies overriding parental rights and the child's autonomy in deciding to live in Turkey. In Turkey, officially it would seem that the girl is regarded as not legally able to marry, but the practice is so common (and presumably regarded as harmless) that no action is usually necessary. Within the rural community in which the girl married, the practice appears to be regarded as not just harmless, but normal. Can UK definitions of what is harmful be applied outside the UK, even to a UK citizen, if that citizen has opted to live in a community with different definitions, and over which the UK has no jurisdiction? If the answer to the above question is no, then the question arises as to whether such definitions can be applied to UK citizens who have opted to live in a community with different values within the UK, provided that no UK laws are broken.

From the viewpoint of the Hasidim, a beneficial act is one that facilitates the advent of the Messiah. Since the Messiah will only come if all Jews keep all of the Laws all of the time, any act, however temporarily effective, such as genetic counselling or fertility limitation, which militates against keeping the Law cannot be of benefit. Any such act which is therefore not beneficial indeed causes harm. However, not all acts which break the Law are necessarily maleficent. For example, all of the Laws can be broken in order to save a life except those relating to idolatry, adultery and murder. Even among the other Laws there are differences. To refrain from breaking a 'Thou shalt not' Law, the whole of one's fortune must be spent. To comply with a 'Thou shalt' Law, only a fifth of one's fortune need be used (Office of the Chief Rabbi, personal communication). On the other hand, no harm can result from keeping the Law. If harm apparently comes to someone as a result of keeping the Law, it would have been within the plan of God, and therefore is not harmful. Thus needs for education or management to secure people's future well-being are needs that will be met if God wills this. Harm cannot therefore accrue if the needs are not met, particularly if to meet them would conflict with observance of the Law. This is borne out in the attitude to disability among Hasidic Jews in Israel, where a significant proportion of parents were found to have no interest in the impact of education on the future of their disabled children, since this was not within their province of concern.[14] The implication of this is that the well-being of the community is all-important, since the welfare of the individual is not only subservient to it, but also dependent on it. For the religious Jew, the coming of the Messiah is the event that will benefit every human being, Jew and Gentile alike, so that any act which hinders the Messiah's coming must cause cosmic harm which transient personal gain or loss cannot counter.

The opposing argument – that the prevention of harm to the individual is paramount, even if this results in wider harm to the entire community – can be illustrated, for example, by Harriet Harman's decision about the education of her son. As a member not only of the British Labour Party, but also at that time of the Shadow Cabinet, she had perforce agreed to and accepted the Party's policy on education – that selection for entry to particular schools is harmful not only to particular children, but is also generally harmful to society at large by creating divisions within that society. Nevertheless, she opted to send her own son to a State school that selects its very academically able pupils. She defended this decision by claiming that her son would be personally benefited by that school and personally harmed by having to go to a local school of low standard. If she stood by her political principles, she would harm her son specifically, whereas if she did not, she might theoretically harm many other children.[15]

This raises the question of whether anyone is justified in causing definite and specific harm to an individual, either himself or another, in order to prevent theoretical harm to a community by, for example, flouting its religious beliefs. For example, a woman in labour had placenta praevia (i.e. the placenta was completely obstructing the exit from the womb). The baby could only be delivered by Caesarean section. The mother was a Jehovah's Witness and had refused blood transfusion. She told me that if I gave her blood it would be a sin on my conscience, not hers. Despite receiving a transfusion, she lost her uterus and the baby died. Had her anaemia been corrected before operation, it is highly likely that the baby would have survived. The death of this baby is therefore directly attributable to the mother's religious belief. There are two questions to be answered here. First, does one ever have the right to make a decision to do something that has a high likelihood of causing harm? Secondly, what is the status of the unborn baby? The first question is of course complex, since it involves not only the decision but also the motive. For example, in a recent television programme,[16] a Royal Air Force officer, having narrowly escaped death while attempting to rescue the crew of a blazing tanker, was winched aboard it again to complete the rescue. This was an action taken in the knowledge that it could have resulted in death or injury to the officer himself, but which was justified by the altruism involved. The medical case seems rather different. The patient took the decision not to have a blood transfusion in the knowledge that although it might result in death or injury to herself and her baby, it would preserve her immortal soul, whereas accepting the transfusion would destroy it. From her point of view, therefore, to die was the lesser evil. Since the transfused blood would not have entered the body of the unborn child, it gained no benefit from the mother's abstinence, but was greatly harmed – the baby died. The RAF officer risked his own life in order to save others, whereas the mother risked her baby's life in order to save herself. Again, in accepting her transference of the decision to me, and giving her the transfusion, I had by my beliefs benefited her by saving her life, but had knowingly destroying her immortal soul according to her beliefs, since even involuntary acceptance of blood has that effect. I had therefore harmed her beyond recall without influencing the fate of the baby.

Drew discusses the management of the pregnant Jehovah's Witness, and is quite clear about his opinion: 'For a doctor . . . to force a patient to have treatment is both morally and legally wrong'.[17] However, he does concede that in cases where a parent is taking the decision for an incompetent minor, things are much less clear-cut: 'and adequate legal provisions [must] exist to protect the child against potentially dangerous views'.[17] The point which he does not address is precisely the problem that the management of pregnant women involves, namely the treatment of two patients – the mother and the unborn child. In my case, the harm done to the baby is clear-cut – he died. However, the relative harm caused by being ostracised from one's community, or receiving less than optimum management of disability, is not so clear-cut.

This type of situation is beautifully analysed in Chaim Potok's novel, *The Gift of Asher Lev*.[18] Asher Lev is a devout Hasidic Jew and a gifted painter. His father is the natural successor to the very old but childless Rebbe, but his appointment as heir apparent is blocked because it is unthinkable that he should be succeeded by Asher, who has offended the whole community with his paintings using the theme of the crucifixion to express the suffering of the Jews. Asher deliberately dissociates himself from his family and the community, and in so doing leaves his own son to succeed his father. In this albeit fictional example, Asher risks his own soul and the integrity and immediate well-being of his family for the good of the community. This is certainly the reverse of the Harriet Harman and Jehovah's Witness examples.

In discussing the management of leukaemia in the children of Jehovah's Witnesses, Kearney emphasises the need to come to a compromise which allows adequate if less than optimum treatment. This is achieved by avoiding blood transfusion, thereby preventing the family disruption that this would cause, the long-term good outweighing the potential short-term harm.[19]

The problem therefore is this. If one is attempting to provide the best possible care for disabled children in communities such as the Hasidim, the two extreme positions both have the potential for harm. At one extreme, providing treatment but only within the system available to all children, so that no note can be taken of religious needs, risks the family being ostracised from their culture and community with the attendant harm that this has the potential to cause. The other extreme, where the religious needs of the family are paramount and must be respected even if this means that no treatment can be provided, results in the children having no opportunity to develop skills which will enable them to live as full a life as they are capable of. The best resolution of this problem may be to take a position between the extremes which produces a balance of harms and which will inevitably require concessions on both sides. The religious community will need to comply with those laws and regulations which do not conflict with the religious needs, in return for the host community complying with those religious requirements that are consistent with adequate treatment.

Such a compromise is not always easy. To what extent can anyone be held responsible for causing harm by an act which is only peripheral to the harm, and which is carried out in the expectation that no harm would occur, but which is done in an attempt to comply with requirements which arise from the family's religious beliefs? For example, I have been asked to provide written evidence not that a daughter does not have a familial disorder, but that my investigations have failed to show that she does. There is therefore the hypothetical risk of harm to the siblings and their partners as a direct result of the parental religious beliefs and my collusion with them. Similarly, a family in which several boys had fragile X syndrome (a genetically determined form of mental retardation) refused to allow an affected daughter to be counselled until after she was married, and had presumably given birth to an affected son. This represents a more extreme example of the foregoing risk of harm since, as the daughter is likely to have many children, the probability of one or more of them being affected must be almost 100%. However, this is not straightforward. Which is the greater harm? Is it more harmful to produce a child similar to her brothers and acceptable within the family already, or to render her incapable of fulfilling her primary role within her community, the role of a wife and mother?

Feinberg questions whether, for example, not telling the daughter restricts her freedom of choice,[2] and he differentiates between a lament based on a platitude, that unalterable physical constraints limit freedom, and constraints to freedom from external factors that could be altered. To say that my Y-chromosomes deprive me of the freedom to be female would illustrate the former, and the chemical conditioning of the test-tube babies in Huxley's *Brave New World* would illustrate the latter. If they were able to, the Epsilons would lament their lack of intelligence resulting from the chemicals added to their nutrients during gestation as being a restriction on their freedom. However, can one restrict one's own freedom? For example, can the deliberate decision to accept a loss of opportunity by lack of secular education in order to conform to an external regime be seen as a restriction of freedom and therefore harmful? Feinberg addresses the question of self-inflicted harm, asking whether it is ever justified for the State to coerce a person into refraining from self-harm.[2] He rejects the views that protecting a person from him- or herself is either never or always a valid ground for coercion, so that a decision has to be made as to when it is a valid ground. He further differentiates between deliberate acts, the desired end of which is to cause self-harm (e.g. knowingly swallowing poison), and acts which are undertaken for another reason, but which greatly increase the risk of self-harm (e.g. heavy smoking). This is in turn affected by the reasonableness or otherwise of the risk. This is not to say that one should always take the most prudent course of action. For example, it may be imprudent for a man who is recovering from a heart attack to work hard to achieve a great end, and thereby risk shortening his life, but it is not necessarily unreasonable. Feinberg defines five considerations in assessing the risk, namely 'the degree of probability that harm to oneself will result from a given course of action', 'the seriousness of the harm being risked', 'the degree of probability that the goal inclining one to shoulder the risk will in fact result from the course of action', 'the value and importance of achieving that goal' and 'the availability or absence of alternative less risky means to the desired goal'.[2] As he claims, a cost-benefit analysis on the above lines would only warrant state intervention if the risk was extreme and unreasonable. He makes a final distinction 'between fully voluntary and not fully voluntary assumptions of risk. One assumes a risk in a fully voluntary way when one shoulders it while informed of all relevant facts and contingencies, and in the absence of all coercive pressure and compulsion'.[2]

How would such a cost–benefit analysis work out when considering the problem of harm in, say, the Hasidic population? This question only arises because there is a potential conflict between maintaining the requirements of the religion and providing adequate therapy for the disabled child. From the viewpoint of the community, the all-important goal to be achieved is the keeping of the Law, and in their opinion this goal is best achieved by maintaining the strict religious schooling. The risk taken is that the child will receive less than adequate treatment. This risk arises because much of the therapy has to be incorporated into the daily living activities of the child. It is not sufficient for the child to receive intermittent therapy sessions in the clinic. This has two consequences. Because, for example, most therapists are female and the people working in a Hasidic school for boys must be male, the therapist may not be acceptable to the school, so that either another therapist has to be diverted to that work, or an additional therapist who is acceptable has to be employed. If the children go to secular schools, although this might achieve the goal of adequate therapy, it would defeat the goal of keeping the Law. One secondary problem is knowing how fully voluntary the decision is, since it could be argued that there is coercive pressure to conform, even on the adults, let alone the children, from the religious community. Furthermore, if a therapist is diverted to work in a number of different schools, the time involved may mean that time spent on other children has to be cut. There are therefore two forms of burden on the wider community here – on the taxpayer generally to fund a benefit that is made necessary by what is not perceived as a general need, and on other disabled children to forego a level of therapy that they would otherwise enjoy in order to accommodate the perceived needs of the Hasidic children. Failure to provide the therapy will deprive the Hasidic children of the means of optimum functioning, and therefore could be viewed as harming them. Insisting that the therapy should be provided in a way and in a place that offends their religious beliefs and so potentially alienates them from their community and their God also harms them if it is accepted that to belong to a community and a family is a benefit, the loss of which can also be regarded as harm. Failure to provide the therapy could not in these terms be seen as a mere non-benefit, but as a definite harm which the State has a duty to prevent. On the other hand, providing such additional levels of therapy from a finite pool does diminish the absolute level of therapy available to other disabled children. Thus for the individual non-Hasidic disabled child, accommodating the perceived needs of the Hasidic children potentially results in a loss of therapy. Since it is claimed that therapy is a benefit, to be deprived of even part of it constitutes harm. There is therefore a conflict of harm. In trying to achieve a balance, the five principles defined by Feingold above can be invoked, since for the Hasidic child to forego therapy in order not to offend the precepts of the religion (whether or not this can be seen as fully voluntary) can be regarded as harm, inflicted on oneself, albeit by the proxy of the parent acting as the agent of the religion. Whether taking the risk of this self-harm is justified depends on the weight that is given to the fourth criterion, namely whether the perceived value of the goal justifies the risk of self-harm. It has been suggested above that the taxpayer may be coerced into providing education for others on the grounds that to be deprived of knowledge of the world is a harm comparable to being deprived of food. If this is so, can it not also be claimed that to provide an education which is so restricted that it also deprives the child of knowledge of the world is equally to harm the child, so that the same argument would apply? The Hasidim can be coerced by this argument into giving their children a broad education that prevents this particular harm. In practical terms this would mean subjecting their schools to inspection and providing an education which conforms to the National Curriculum, in addition to the religious education. Therefore in attempting to decide whether the goal is worth the risk attendant on achieving it, four harms have to be balanced, namely alienation from the community if the children are required to attend a secular school, suboptimal functioning if therapy is not provided, harm to other disabled children if finite resources are diverted, and harm to the Hasidic children due to depriving them of a balanced education if the State colludes with a restricted education. This balance will be largely subjective, depending on the weight that is attached to the four harms.

The provision of potentially compromised therapy for Hasidic children in order not to compromise their own or their parents' religious beliefs may involve the physician or therapist in compromising his or her own beliefs – that is, in colluding with less than adequate therapy. This may harm the interests of the therapist.

References

1 Sykes JB (ed.) (1976) *Concise Oxford Dictionary* (6e). Oxford University Press, Oxford.

2 Feinberg J (1973) *Social Philosophy*. Prentice-Hall Inc., Englewood Cliffs, NJ, pp. 9, 25, 30, 31, 47, 48.

3 Jones RB (1993) An evaluation of the character of the moral debate about abortion. *Eur J Pub Health*. 3: 141–5.

4 Beauchamp TL and Childress JE (1983) *Principles of Biomedical Ethics* (2e). Oxford University Press, New York, p. 109.

5 Daniels N (1981) Health-care needs and distributive justice. In: M Cohen, T Nagel and T Scanlon (eds) *Medicine and Moral Philosophy*. Princeton University Press, Princeton, NJ, pp. 81–114.

6 Wiggins D and Derman S (1987) Needs, need, needing. *J Med Ethics*. 13: 62–8.

7 Willard LD (1982) Needs and medicine. *J Med Phil*. 7: 259–74.

8 Acheson RM (1978) The definition and identification of need for health care. *J Epidemiol Commun Health*. 32: 10–15.

9 Moore D (1990) The limits of health care. In: D Evans (ed.) *Why Should We Care?* Macmillan Press, London, pp. 75–84.

10 *Education Act 1981*. HMSO, London.

11 World Health Organization (1980) *International Classification of Impairments, Disabilities and Handicaps*. World Health Organization, Geneva, p. 183.

12 Newman LE (1992) Jewish theology and bioethics. *J Med Phil.* **17**: 309–27.

13 Sacks J (1990) The 1990 Reith Lectures. 3. The family. *Listener.* **124**: 16–18.

14 Leyser Y and Dekel G (1991) Perceived stress and adjustment in religious Jewish families with a child who is disabled. *J Psychol.* **125**: 427–38.

15 Hoggert S (1994) Policy and politics. Sketch: Patten gives Labour end-of-term lesson. *The Guardian.* **6 December**: 8.

16 BBC Television (1996) *999 Special.* Broadcast on 8/10/96.

17 Drew NC (1981) The pregnant Jehovah's Witness. *J Med Ethics.* **7**: 137–9.

18 Potok C (1990) *The Gift of Asher Lev.* William Heinemann Ltd, London.

19 Kearney PJ (1978) Leukaemia in children of Jehovah's Witnesses: issues and priorities in a conflict of care. *J Med Ethics.* **4**: 32–5.

Chapter 6

The interests and rights of the patient

A patient who enters treatment can expect that her interests will be recognised, and that this is a duty of the physician. It is the patient's right. As Waldron puts it, in relation to free speech, '[that this] is understood in terms of recognition that an individual's interest . . . is a sufficient ground for holding other individuals and agencies to be under duties of various sorts'.[1]

There are two aspects to the patient's interest, namely the general and the medical aspect. In general terms it is necessary for this to be holistic – the patient being considered as a whole person existing within a family and society. This is particularly relevant for members of a religious society, since it may influence the acceptance of the medical aspects of treatment. From the medical point of view it is in the patient's interest that an accurate diagnosis is made, that the treatment is appropriate, that it carries an appropriate risk for the benefit obtained, and that the patient is fully informed about the treatment and has given his or her full informed consent to it. This consent issue is complicated if the patient is a child. It must take into account when they should be deemed able to understand the information presented and consent to it. These two things may not necessarily be coincident. A further complication which arises in strict religious groups is that, even for adults, no store is placed on personal autonomy if the exercise of this conflicts with the religion, while the autonomy of children is often further restricted by the need for total obedience to the parent.

At what point is the child competent to speak for him- or herself? And until that time, who speaks for him – the parent or the professional? In one religion, Judaism, this may seem to be an easy decision. The boy becomes bar mitzvah, and therefore adult, on his thirteenth birthday, and the girl becomes bat mitzvah on her twelfth birthday, so presumably at this point they become competent to take the same autonomous decisions that can be made by any adult.

Feldman questions this. He points out that the suffix '-escent' implies a growing or developing, and that although becoming bar or bat mitzvah brings responsibilities, these are not complete until the age of 20 years, when the adolescent becomes baronshin or batonshin – responsible enough to be punished.[2] Until that time there is a two-way responsibility that is enshrined in the sixth commandment: 'Honour thy father and thy mother, that thy days may be long upon the land which the Lord thy God giveth thee (Exodus, Chapter 20, verse 12). He notes the father's prayer at the son's bar mitzvah: 'Thank God for removing responsibility for this child from me'. Halakhic sources interpret this as meaning the responsibility for educating the son, which passes from the father to the son at bar mitzvah. This is a most important ruling, since part of the problem of providing adequate treatment for these children is the need for them to be educated in religious schools. However, parental responsibility for the moral and spiritual well-being of the adolescent remains, and the parents have a right to information to allow them to judge whether an action (e.g. the taking of contraceptives) is compatible with that well-being. However, if in the opinion of the doctor or social worker the disclosure of information to the parents about the adolescent's medical history would alienate the adolescent further from benign influence and care, then disclosure should not take place. There is no suggestion that the adolescent should decide on disclosure. Adults are said to need to know the adolescents, and therefore presumably also the children, well enough to take the decision on disclosure for them. Clearly the child has no part to play in deciding on his or her own best interests. A corollary of this is that a child need never be asked to give consent, since adults know best what is in the child's interest. It is also implicit that, although the children become ritually adult at bar mitzvah and bat mitzvah, they are not considered to be truly adult in the sense of being able to make their own decisions about giving or withholding consent.

Jakobovits implies further that, where life-saving treatment is concerned, consent is not needed from adults or children, since it would offend Jewish law for a doctor to refuse to give treatment without consent, given that the overriding duty of the doctor is to preserve life.[3] Since it is also the duty of the patient to have his or her life preserved, withholding consent in these circumstances would also presumably offend Jewish law. The duty is absolute, based on the claim that the body is the property of God, not of the person occupying it. No mention is made of whether non-life-preserving treatment (e.g. the management of disability) can be given without consent. However, in secular medical practice, it is accepted that informed consent to treatment is required.

Jakobovits claims that for a doctor to insist on informed consent can, in some circumstances, constitute a failure of professional duty by the doctor.[3] He cites the example of a patient who is told about three possible treatments, and is then asked to decide which one he wants to receive. This, he claims, is a case of the doctor abrogating his responsibility to exercise the skill and knowledge that he possesses, and thereby putting unwarranted stress on the patient. If this was what was involved in seeking informed consent, then he would be right. In my view, however, informed consent gives the patient the opportunity to accept or reject the advice of the doctor on the basis of information rather than ignorance. It does not absolve the doctor from the responsibility of advising the patient on what he considers to be the best treatment, nor is it in the patient's interest that he do so.

Jakobovits places a duty on the physician to lie rather than be open about the diagnosis and prognosis, if in his opinion there is the slightest chance that telling the truth would cause distress or destroy hope. He bases this on the passage in 2 Kings, Chapter 8, verse 10, in which Elisha says to the messenger of the king of Syria, 'Go say unto him, thou mayest certainly recover: howbeit the Lord hath shewed me that he shall surely die'. However, as Levin[4] points out,[4] there is contrary advice, to be brutally frank, in 2 Kings, Chapter 20, verse 1: 'give your last instructions to your household, for you are a dying man and will not recover'.[7] This paternalistic attitude – that those in authority know better what is in the patient's interest than he does himself, is not confined to one particular interpretation of Jewish law. It even has a role in British law. An editorial commenting on a case involving informed consent points out that even though the decision was that the doctor should disclose any risk inherent in a treatment which was a material risk in the sense that 'a reasonable patient . . . would be likely to attach significance to the risk . . . in determining whether or not to forego the proposed therapy', the doctor need not disclose the risk if 'reasonable medical assessment indicated that disclosure would pose a serious threat to the health of the patient'.[5] Redmon takes the opposite view on consent to be used in research.[6] He quotes the New York Board of Regents, saying that 'no consent is valid unless it is . . . based on a disclosure of all material facts. Any fact which might influence the giving or withholding of consent is material'. In suggesting that the researcher does not even have the doctor's relationship with the patient, and therefore 'no basis for the exercise of the usual professional judgement' as to whether information should be withheld, he does however support the idea that a treating doctor can in certain circumstances withhold information from a patient. If informed consent is to have any meaning, it must mean that the patient is fully informed. So-called 'informed consent' that is based on partial information, however well intentioned, is not informed consent.

Much of the medical literature on informed consent is concerned with either valid consent to research, or refusal of life-saving treatment by the parents of a child patient. There is little on the less dramatic problem of whether a child has a right to an opinion on the everyday, non-life-saving management of, for example, disability. However, in a feature on the welfare of children and young people in hospital, Alderson points out that one of the ten required standards states that 'The consent *of the child* and the parent or guardian should be obtained to treat children under age 16, save in an emergency'.[7] The emphasis is mine, but the order – child before parent – is theirs. The article goes on to say that even in the case of children who are too young to consent, their wishes should be ascertained, and that for older children parental consent is not essential. Alderson quotes the 'Gillick' judgement,[8] which states that parents lose the right of consent for children under 16 years of age, 'if and when the child achieves a sufficient understanding and intelligence to enable him or her fully to understand what is proposed'.[7] This only applies if the child is consenting to proposed treatment. Dickenson cites case law that denies children (in England and Wales at least) the right to refuse treatment.[9] The child is in the incongruous position of being able to give consent without having the corollary right to withhold it, which of course throws doubt on the whole idea that they can give consent at all. This incongruity is confirmed by the Medical Defence Union,[10] which cites (as does Dickenson) the case of a girl with anorexia nervosa under the age of 16 years who refused to give her consent to forcible feeding. She was overruled by the judge at the request of her parents and the health authority, even though she was Gillick competent.[11] The conclusion is that if a child under 16 years of age refuses treatment and the parents consent to it, this allows the doctor to proceed, but it does not *require* him to do so. This is a further instance where consent from both the child and the parent can be overruled, since the decision as to whether treatment should proceed or not is the doctor's. In Scottish law the situation is different. According to the Age of Legal Capacity (Scotland) Act 1991, the age of consent is 16 years, and 'a person under the age of sixteen shall have legal capacity to consent on his own behalf . . . where, in the opinion of a qualified medical practitioner attending him, he is capable of understanding the nature and possible consequences of the procedure or treatment'.[12] McConnell interprets this as meaning that consent encompasses agreement to and refusal of treatment, and argues that there is no real right to consent if the child is not allowed to make a decision which is objectively unreasonable, and against his or her own best interest. However, it does again give the overriding decision to the physician. As Alderson points out,[7] consent is only valid in any case if the patient is fully informed, which involves the information being presented in a form that is appropriate to the development of the receiver. An editorial announcing the setting up of a working party to study the ethics of research on children comments on the confusion in the codes of conduct.[13] The Declaration of Helsinki requires all research subjects to be volunteers, and the Nuremberg Code requires that they have the legal capacity to give consent, free power of choice and sufficient knowledge to make such a choice. It points out that the Medical Research Council is quite specific: 'parents . . . cannot give consent on their [the children's] behalf to any procedures which are of no particular benefit to them and which may carry some risk of harm'. By 1980, the British Paediatric Association had stated that a cost–benefit analysis could justify research on children, even in cases where the risk to the child was more than negligible, if there was great benefit to society. In the revision of their document they have three categories of risk – minimal, low and high – and they state that it is unethical to submit children to more than minimal risk if the procedure offers them no personal benefit. However, they also state that 'research that is of no intended benefit to the child subject is not necessarily unethical or illegal'.[14]

What level of maturity is necessary for children and adolescents to give valid consent, and how can this be assessed? Koren *et al.* propose the babysitter test.[15] Canada and the USA have nationally validated courses on babysitting for children from 10 to 12 years of age. This implies that these children have sufficient maturity not only to cope with the everyday tasks of, for example, feeding a baby, but also to deal with potentially life-threatening situations. However, these same children are deemed at best to be capable of assenting to consent that is given by their parents. Koren *et al.*[15] quote McCormick, who suggests that since if they are capable, children would want to consent to procedures in the same way that their parents consent for them, because they ought to, proxy consent is valid.[16] Ramsey[17] claims that McCormick treats children as small adults. In fact, in his introductory paragraph McCormick states that, pharmacologically at any rate, they 'are not to be regarded simply as little people'.[16] He is claiming that there are certain things that we ought to do, and others which are over and above what we ought to do, which are in effect acts of charity that are dependent on grace rather than duty. The former 'are . . . identifiable values that we ought to support . . . because they are definitive of our flourishing and well-being'.[16] He sees participation in research that is of no personal benefit, but which is of benefit to society, without posing significant risk to ourselves, as one of these values. Therefore even if a child is too young to give their valid consent to such participation, parental proxy consent is valid, because were the child able to consent he or she ought to, and would therefore want to do so. This implies that everyone wants to do what they ought to do – a claim which is difficult to justify. However, it could be argued that if it is truly definitive of everyone's flourishing and well-being, this would include the child, and therefore it would be in their best interest, too.

Ramsey defends his own position by claiming that McCormick does treat children as small adults whose moral responsibilities are discharged by the proxy of their parents, since they would agree if they were adults. He quotes from his book *The Patient as Person*: 'To attempt to consent for a child to be made an experimental subject is to treat a child as not a child. It is to treat him as if he were an adult person who has consented. . . . If the grounds for this are alleged to be the presumptive or implied consent of the child, that must simply be characterised as a violent and a false presumption.'[17] He seems to be claiming that consent can never be given by another for a child to be an experimental subject, regardless of the level of risk to the child, without violating the Kantian imperative always to use a person as an end rather than just as a means. On the other hand, he argues that if it is imperative to conduct research on children if paediatric medicine is to progress, then we have to appeal to the doctrine of the lesser of two evils: 'Either way they do wrong. It is immoral not to do the research. It is also immoral to use children who cannot themselves consent. . . . On this supposition research medicine . . . is a realm in which men have to "sin bravely".'[17] This avoids the central issue – that the overriding concern in treatment or research programmes must be the interests of the child. No harm must come to the child as a result of the research procedures. This is easy to decide in cases where no invasive procedures are required (e.g. a questionnaire survey) and equally easy in cases where the procedures are so invasive that they clearly cause harm (e.g. administering a drug with known severe side-effects). But how invasive, for example, is a blood test? For some children it is no more than a minor unpleasantness, while for others it is a cause of near terror. In such a case, the welfare of the child rather than the benefit of the research project must be the criterion for judging whether the procedure should be performed, and safeguards must be written into the research protocol to ensure that this is so. Even if it is accepted that proxy consent can be valid for using children as research subjects, this does not absolve the research worker or the parents from taking note of the child's opinions of what is in his or her own interest. Koren *et al.* quote several studies which suggest that at seven years of age children are able to understand the implications of research procedures, but that most societies require them to be 13 or 14 years old before their own consent can override the proxy consent of their carers.[15] They also quote Freedman, who claims that since children are not independent they have no right to be left alone, but only the right to be taken care of. He claims that once risk versus benefit has been considered, proxy consent – and therefore presumably the interests of the child – is not an issue.[18] This sweeping generalisation is out of kilter with other work. Redmon seeks a Kantian solution to the problem of consent by children, and defines four criteria for accepting such consent, namely that 'we can reasonably expect the child to identify with the goals of the research when she is an adult', that 'the identification will be strong enough to outweigh the harm of the knowledge of being used by her parents',[6] that she assents to the procedure if she is old enough to do so, and that the risk is minimal. If these criteria can be fulfilled, then Redmon feels that it can be claimed that the child has been an end, not just a means.

Consent to treatment is less contentious than consent to research, since if the treatment is not in the patient's best interest, it should not be used in any case. However, obtaining consent does hinge on the age at which the child can be deemed to understand enough to take part in the decision. Alderson found evidence of the ability of very young children to understand complex issues in a study in which 120 children who had been admitted for surgery, their parents and medical and other hospital professionals were interviewed.[19] This showed that children as young as 5 years had an understanding of death and could evaluate the significance of proposed treatment, even that as serious as heart–lung transplantation, and that it is possible for adults to evaluate their understanding. Alderson makes the point that if long-term treatment is involved, it has to be with the child's willing consent if compliance is to be obtained. This is particularly relevant to the management of disabled children, because of the invariable long-term nature of this management. Clearly, treatment with which the patient does not comply is of no benefit, and cannot be regarded as being in the interests of anyone – patient, physician or society at large.

However, on the basis of cognitive developmental theory, Grant claims that children who have not reached the stage of formal operations – that is, an ability 'to be able to weigh up the advantages and disadvantages of different suggestions concerning . . . treatment and lifestyle options' – are intrinsically incapable of making a decision for themselves.[20] She claims that this is usually achieved between the ages of 11 and 14 years, and that until then they should be presented with a fait accompli by the doctor and parents acting together. This of course runs counter to Alderson's interpretation of the findings of her study. To back up her assertion, Grant describes the case of a 9-year-old girl with 55% body burns, who refused a temporary graft of pig skin. At this age (the stage of the concrete operational child), it is claimed that children tend to view things as either wholly good or wholly bad, so that it was inappropriate to discuss treatment options with the child. An alternative view might be that far from being unable to decide, this child shared the abhorrence of many people of all ages of the concept of inter-species transplantation. Alternatively, the temporary nature of the graft may not have been made clear, so that the girl believed that she might turn into a pig.

If the child is old enough to express an opinion, however old that is deemed to be, there is at least the potential for his or her views to be taken into account, and for the parent's proxy consent to be over-ridden by them if this is seen to be in the child's best interest. However, if the child is preverbal or prenatal, then the law would need to be invoked with a view to discovering whether 'the child's proper development is being avoidably neglected . . . and also that he is in need of care'.[21]

For Wierenga, the criterion of validity for proxy consent for incompetent patients is the best interest of the patient.[22] By this it is meant not that it need be known to be in the best interest, since there may not be sufficient data to decide this, but that it is believed to be in the best interest. The problem of how to evaluate best interest is addressed by Pardess *et al.* in the different context of deciding the best interest of the child when preparing expert testimony in medico-legal cases involving abuse or custody.[23] They feel that this is best carried out by a team, which is separate from and independent of the team that is treating the child. This has the following advantages:

- *it enhances validity and reliability*
- *it reduces bias due to subjective beliefs and values*
- *it serves as a source of sharing and support*
- *interdisciplinary teamwork enables the integration of different theoretical models and the use of various techniques and examinations.*[23]

Up to this point I have only considered the interests of the patient in terms of the application of medical interventions. However, the patient, child or adult, is not 'a case of Down syndrome' or 'one of the mentally handicapped' or 'a spastic'. He or she is a person with a family, with wider relationships both within and without his or her own community, who *among other things* has Down syndrome or whatever. This requires a holistic approach to treatment and the interests and rights that accrue from it. It is an unfortunate feature of paediatric medical practice that it is not invariably in the child's interest to maintain the family bond. If the child is being physically or sexually abused, it is relatively straightforward to accept that this is so. It is also relatively easy to accept that if the family refuses to give consent to any medical intervention that is necessary to save the child's life, the law should be invoked. However, religious families rarely refuse to allow an intervention, but acknowledging the very existence of disability may have far-reaching consequences for such a family, ranging from a theoretical taint of lawlessness associated with the child's conception to the very practical difficulties of finding partners for the siblings. To accept treatment does involve acknowledging the disability, and can influence the parents' willingness to give consent. Even when the difficulties are not so extreme, problems may arise because the requirements of the family and of the group may mean that the treatment cannot be provided in the most convenient place for the therapist, or with the intensity necessary to achieve an optimum effect. Therefore a conflict of interests can arise, because it is in the interest of the child that they receive adequate treatment, and it is also in their interest that they are not alienated from their family and society. This leads to a second conflict – between the interests of the child and the interests of the host community and the resources that it has to offer to all of its members if a disproportionate amount of those resources is diverted to meet the specific needs of these families.

To summarise, therefore, if the interests of the patient are to be safeguarded, two aspects of care must be considered. First, from a purely medical standpoint, the treatment must be appropriate to the condition that is being treated. It must be capable of achieving a defined and beneficial result. Any harm which results from the treatment must be appropriate to the benefit received. The patient must be fully informed about the treatment and any suitable alternatives. In the case of a child, their views must be sought at a level appropriate to their development. If the child is not mature enough to understand the treatment and give consent to it, it is in their interest that this is undertaken by an appropriate agent. This will usually, but not invariably, be the parents.

Secondly, from a wider viewpoint, it is usually in the patient's interest, particularly if he or she is a child, that the integrity of the family is maintained, and that as far as possible the family is able to maintain its own lifestyle within its chosen community. The dilemma is that these two elements of the child's interest may not be compatible. In this situation, either the physician (and, through him or her, the host community) may have to accept a suboptimal level of treatment in order to satisfy this second wider interest, or the parents and the minority community may have to compromise in order to achieve adequate therapy for the child.

References

1 Waldron J (1984) Introduction. In: J Waldron (ed.) *Theories of Rights.* Oxford University Press, Oxford, pp. 1–20.

2 Feldman DM (1984) Rabbinic comment: the rights of adolescents. *Mt Sinai J Med.* **51**: 49–51.

3 Jakobovits I (1989) Some Jewish teaching on doctor/patient relationships. *Med- Leg J.* **57**: 19–33.

4 Levin S (1973) Jewish ethics in relation to medicine. *S Afr Med J.* **47**: 924–30.

5 Anon (1985) Adequately informed consent. *J Med Ethics.* **11**: 115–16.

6 Redmon RB (1986) How children can still be respected as 'ends' yet still be used as subjects in non-therapeutic research. *J Med Ethics.* **12**: 77–82.

7 Alderson P (1991) Out of the darkness. *Health Serv J.* **3 October**: 22–4.

8 Gillick v West Norfolk & Wisbech AHA (1985) 3 *All ER* 402–37.

9 Dickenson D (1994) Children's informed consent to treatment: is the law an ass? *J Med Ethics.* **20**: 205–6.

10 Gilberthorpe J (1997) *Consent to Treatment.* Medical Defence Union Ltd, London.

11 ReW (a minor) (1992) 4 *All ER* 627.

12 McConnell AA (1995) Children's informed consent to treatment: the Scottish dimension. *J Med Ethics.* **21**: 186–7.

13 Anon (1982) Clinical research on children (editorial). *J Med Ethics.* **8**: 3–4.

14 British Paediatric Association (1992) *Guidelines for the Ethical Conduct of Medical Research Involving Children.* British Paediatric Association, London.

15 Koren G, Carmeli DB, Carmeli YS and Haslam R (1993) Maturity of children to consent to medical research: the babysitter test. *J Med Ethics.* **19**: 142–7.

16 McCormick RS (1974) Proxy consent in the experimentation situation. *Perspect Biol Med.* **18**: 2–20.

17 Ramsey P (1976) The enforcement of morals: non-therapeutic research on children. *Hastings Cent Rep.* **6**: 21–30.

18 Freedman B (1979) A moral theory of informed consent. *Hastings Cent Rep.* **5**: 32–9.

19 Alderson P (1992) In the genes or in the stars? Children's competence to consent. *J Med Ethics.* **18**: 119–24.

20 Grant VJ (1991) Consent in paediatrics: a complex teaching assignment. *J Med Ethics.* **17**: 199–204.

21 *Children and Young Persons Act 1969*. Part 1. Subsection 1(2). HMSO, London.

22 Wierenga E (1983) Proxy consent and counterfactual wishes. *J Med Phil.* **8**: 405–16.

23 Pardess E, Finzi R and Sever J (1993) Evaluating the best interest of the child – a model of multidisciplinary teamwork. *Med Law.* **12**: 205–11.

Chapter 7

The interests and rights of the parents

The interests of parents within the context of the medical and educational management of their child are complicated, since the interests of each of the other agents that are involved impinge on them. In that they are acting as locum patients, their interests and those of the patient coincide, so that the decisions that they take on behalf of the child should be in his or her best interest, the difficulty being to define what that is. This may not be the same as what would be in their best interest were they themselves the patient. In addition, the child and their parents are all members of the same family, and it is usually in all of their interests to maintain the integrity of that family. In religious communities the children often also have an obligation to honour and obey their parents in all things (Exodus, Chapter 20, verse 12). The interests of a particular sect may also impinge, so a conflict of interests could arise. For example, if the religion demanded that the child attend a religious school, but the treatment of the child would be better served by their going to a secular school, the parents might not choose the latter option.

The role of the parent is not just that of a concerned adult – it is that of the concerned adult who is normally regarded as being responsible for safeguarding all aspects of the child's welfare, and taking decisions about management, sometimes in opposition to others such as the physician or the child. Who makes the decision when the wishes of the child and the parents do not coincide? Is it the parents, the physician, society or the child himself?

If it is the parents' right, and therefore in their interest, to act as a proxy for their child, this needs to be clarified, since the whole concept of proxy consent is unclear and may itself be misleading. Vandeveer quotes a report of the National Commission for the Protection of Human Subjects of Biomedical and Behavioural Research, which distinguishes between what can be done autonomously, consent, and what can be done on behalf of another, giving permission.[1] He points out that the normal meaning of the word 'proxy' is one who has been empowered to act for another person *by that person*, and that this is manifestly not the case for children. He dismisses McCormick's contention that children can be assumed to want to consent to such research, because they ought to,[2] on the grounds that the children having not voluntarily partaken of the benefits of the research, have no duty to contribute to it, although McCormick's position is that there is a duty to take part in research which poses no harm to oneself, even if no personal benefit accrues from participation. This argument hangs on the definition of proxy. Can a person act as another's proxy without that person's knowledge and consent? There are two dictionary definitions of proxy, namely 'agency of a substitute or deputy' and 'person authorised to act for another'.[3] What is not clear is who can authorise in this way. The examples that are given for the first definition (voted, or was married, by proxy) do imply consent from the person assigning the proxy. On the other hand, the example given for the second definition (stood proxy for the grandmother) does not necessarily do so, if, for example, the reason why the grandmother herself could not attend was that she was demented. In the same dictionary the definition does not make it clear whether consent can be given for another. However, a second dictionary uses only examples which imply the need for consent from the person appointing the proxy.[4] Clearly if a child can appoint a proxy, he or she does not need one.

If one moves from consent to permission, does this alter the power of the person giving the permission? Is there any need in either case for the best interests of the child to be taken into account? If, for example, I am moving from a house with a garden to a third-floor flat without one, the decision to have my dog put down is one to which I can consent without regard to the best interests of the dog, unless death is in the better interest of the dog than life in a flat. To say that I give permission for the dog to be put down in no way alters the situation, although the *Oxford English Dictionary* suggests that consent, derived from the Latin 'con' and 'sentire' (to feel together, to agree), implies that the person agrees with that to which he is consenting – there is a consensus. Permission does not necessarily imply agreement. One definition that is given, for example, is 'fail to prevent'.

It is necessary to differentiate between three ideas. First, for a parent to give proxy consent implies that they have a mandate from the child to take the decision, knowing what he or she would decide, and given that he or she would be capable of deciding. Secondly, to give consent implies that they are in agreement with what is proposed and have the right to decide for the child. Thirdly, to give permission implies only that they allow a procedure, possibly without themselves agreeing with it (e.g. a Jehovah's Witness who allows her child to have a blood transfusion). The first option is redundant, since if it applied, the child would not need it.

Vandeveer points out that, even in decisions that are clearly in the child's best interest, for example, the application of life-saving treatment, we often cannot be said to have the child's consent.[1] How then can the child's best interest be constructed, and by whom? Seeking parental consent rests on two assumptions – first, that the interests of the child have moral importance, and secondly, that the parents are the people who have the right to decide.

This can perhaps be clarified by considering one class of patient in whom it will never be possible to obtain consent, namely the patient in an irreversible permanent vegetative state, whose organs are required for transplantation, and whose views on the matter are not known. Current practice is that, once dead, such a patient's organs can be used with the consent of the next-of-kin. A recent case has brought this into sharp focus. Doctors caring for a man who was comatose and dying were asked by his wife to obtain semen which could be stored and used after his death to impregnate her. This was done, but permission to use the semen was denied by the courts on the grounds that written consent was required from the donor for any gametes to be used in this way. Here proxy in the sense of someone representing the demented grandmother was not accepted. It was further argued that this post-mortem use of 'donor organs' was qualitatively different from use of his kidneys, since gametes were taken while he was still alive but unable to consent, but for a purpose that in all other circumstances would require his acquiescence – to create his child. Even though the mother would in this case be his wife, once a precedent was set, this could be extended to use patients in a permanent vegetative state as virtually unlimited gamete donors.

There are two main theories for determining the basis for consenting for another, namely the *substituted judgement test*, which asks what the incompetent person would have wished if they were competent, and the *best interest test*, which asks what would be in the best interest of the incompetent patient. If the word 'proxy' is to be used at all, it can only be used in connection with the substituted judgement test, the implication being that the wishes of the child are in fact known. O'Neil,[5] using the Brother Fox case,[6] points out that in the USA, many states have enacted living-will legislation which distinguishes between an advisory directive, executed before diagnosis, and requiring the physician only to take note of the wishes of the patient, and a binding directive, which is made after diagnosis of a terminal illness and is binding on the physician to withdraw life support.[7] Brother Fox had apparently made no such living will. However, he had made clear on several occasions, including just prior to the surgery that left him in a permanent vegetative state, mainly in discussion of the Karen Quinlan case,[8] that he opposed the use of a respirator in patients in a permanent vegetative state. Despite the lack of a written directive, O'Neil sees this as an incompetent person having made an explicit choice while previously competent. The case of Karen Quinlan is not so clear-cut. The evidence that she did not want extraordinary means used to prolong her life was based on general statements that were made while she was still well, and which although specific were made when there was no thought that they would apply to her. A further problem is that neither of these cases is entirely relevant to children, since they are usually individuals currently deemed to be incompetent, who have the potential to become competent.

O'Neil differentiates between the Brother Fox case and that of Karen Quinlan, in that Brother Fox made his wishes expressly known immediately prior to the onset of incompetency, in the knowledge that he might become incompetent, so that there was, as the court ruled, no question of a substituted judgement, as opposed to merely passing on Brother Fox's own wishes. However, Karen Quinlan had only made her wishes known in general, with no thought that she would become incompetent. Nevertheless, the court accepted the substituted judgement of Karen Quinlan's family. As O'Neil points out, although choices that are remote from the events carry less weight than those which are made contingent on the events, they should be borne in mind when attempting to apply the best interests or the substituted judgement tests. If the views of the patient when competent are not known, or are unknowable, O'Neil argues that the substituted judgement test is inappropriate, and the best interest test should be applied. The problem is how to determine the best interest of the child, since this will depend to a large extent on the views of the proxy, or even on what the proxy would do if he or she were in the same situation. In an attempt to overcome this problem, O'Neil introduces a 'rational choice' standard. What choice would 'a reasonable or rational person make if situated in circumstances *in all ways* similar to those of the incompetent person?'[5] He points out that the best interest test and the rational choice test should yield identical results. He emphasises that this is not the same as asking what a reasonable person would do in this situation. Rather it is asking what this person, given his abilities and disabilities, would do. He cites as an example the case of a demented elderly man who requires kidney dialysis to stay alive. Most people would prefer death to the indignity of dementia, but since this man does not appreciate the indignity by virtue of his dementia, that would not be part of his rational choice.

In the case of children, in applying the rational choice standard, O'Neil accepts that most can be expected to achieve autonomy, and that this is one of their chief interests, and therefore must be taken into account

when making the rational choice. He cites as an example the case of a
two-year-old requiring treatment for leukaemia which has a 50% chance
of success. Since giving the treatment significantly increases the likelihood of the child achieving autonomy, and not giving it virtually
destroys this, the rational choice is to give the treatment, since this is
in the child's best interest.

Even if everyone concerned is in broad agreement about what is
believed to be the best interest, the chosen option does not always
work out. Higgs describes the case of a nine-year-old boy with advanced
bone cancer, whose surgeon colluded with the parents in not telling him
what his condition was, and that a likely treatment was amputation, on
the grounds that he was too young to cope with it. As a result, his
questions to other members of the team could not be answered.[9]
However, even the agreement is typically lacking in some religious
groups. For example, for the Hasidic parent the best interest of everyone,
child and adult alike, is always served by obeying the Law of God, even if
that interferes with what others consider to be proper management of the
disability, whereas for the therapists this is not usually so.

It is the parents' right, and therefore in their interest, to contribute to
decisions on what is in the child's best interest. Do they have a similar
right to make substituted judgements of what the child would do? In the
Brother Fox and Karen Quinlan cases, there was some basis for making
such a judgement because information was available on their previously
stated opinions. At no point has a child been competent to make the
judgement if he or she is deemed too young to make it at the time. For
example, if it is in the interests of the child and the parents to maintain
the integrity of the family, and this is dependent on complying with the
requirements of a particular religious group, can it be assumed that the
child would agree to that compliance? Such compliance could involve
agreement to practices associated with beliefs (usually very strongly
held) which harm those who hold those beliefs. An example would be
the practice of female circumcision. This varies from a relatively minor
operation to remove the prepuce of the clitoris to infibulation, and major
removal of the clitoris and much of the vulva, with almost total closure
of the orifice.[10] Although it is said that this is accepted by and is only
harmful to the recipient, she is often a young girl who may not be
competent to consent at that time. However, women who have been
circumcised as girls usually insist on the orifice being re-closed following childbirth, and they also usually insist on their daughters being
circumcised, so they can be said to agree with the practice. There is little
condemnation of the comparable practice of male circumcision,
although this is usually a medically unnecessary operation that is
performed as part of the initiation rituals by Jews and Muslims.

Abu-Sahlieh, in a criticism from a Muslim viewpoint of both male and female circumcision, argues that both are in fact contrary to the teachings of the Koran, in that they imply that God did not produce a perfect creation in mankind if it has to be altered by man himself.[11] Both are practices hallowed only by long custom, and should therefore come under the stricture of Article 24 of the Convention on the Rights of the Child, which he quotes: 'States . . . shall take all effective and appropriate measures with a view to abolishing traditional practices prejudicial to the health of children'.[11] This is not confined to religious ritual requirements. A recent television programme[12] described major facial surgery on babies with Down syndrome, which was performed so that the child's appearance would conform to society's norms, but with no discernible benefit to the child. I have argued that even consenting to named children appearing on medical programmes on television is something that is of no benefit to the child and is not therefore in the child's interest, and that no one – not even the parent – has the right to consent to it.[13] It is the parents' right, and in their interest, to be involved in decisions on the child patient's best interest, but not to make a substituted judgement on their behalf.

It is in the parents' interest to maintain the integrity of the family, and for families within a strict religious culture it is in their interest that the tenets of this culture be respected. There are two elements to this, their right to hold their beliefs, and their right to act on them. It is with the latter element that problems arise. If the action leads to the child being harmed, then it cannot be said to be in the child's interest, and therefore it is in society's interest to prevent it. In this context I have already discussed genital mutilation as a rite of passage. In my view, for example, facial plastic surgery for children with Down syndrome is similar to this. It is undertaken because of the belief that society will respond differently to the child who looks different.[14] A more generalised form of this concerns beliefs about what constitutes proper chastisement of children. Those who advocate strict discipline often misuse the phrase 'spare the rod and spoil the child', which is actually much more forceful: 'He that spareth his rod hateth his son: but he that loveth him chastiseth him betimes' (Proverbs, Chapter 13, verse 24). This injunction has resulted in behaviour that would now be regarded as child abuse.

Can the beliefs of a minority religious group be accommodated without compromising adequate provision for the needs of disabled children within the group? Can the beliefs of individuals and communities be respected, even if they conflict with the majority view, or put an additional burden on the general community? From the viewpoint of groups such as the Hasidim, there is no doubt that they believe this to be the most essential aspect of care, since anything which conflicts with their beliefs about what is the Law of God must *ipso facto* be harmful.

Must we always respect other people's beliefs? Of more immediate and practical concern, if we must respect their beliefs, does that not imply that we must also accept the results of holding those beliefs? As Bradney comments, to say that I adhere to a particular faith, implies that if my beliefs are respected, my actions based on that belief must also be respected.[15] Is it possible to respect a belief or an action based on a belief without approving of it? Must one always take account of the patient's or parents' beliefs and attempt to act within them when planning treatment? It is possible to respect someone with whom one disagrees. For example, two people can respect each other despite the fact that one does and the other does not believe in God. However, is it possible to respect someone whose beliefs or actions are anathema to you? Must respecting a person's beliefs not imply an acceptance and approval of them as a whole, including their beliefs or actions, even if it does not necessarily imply agreement?

A further question is whether respect is in any way related to interests and rights. If a behaviour affects only the people involved in it, whether that behaviour is, for example, smoking, drug taking or sadomasochism, does the respect or lack of it of the rest of society have any relevance in restricting the rights of the participants? In the case of homosexual acts between consenting adults, this has only recently been resolved in law in the UK, and certainly does not yet receive universal respect from the community. In one particular situation, namely the acceptance of practising homosexuals as Anglican priests, the two opposing arguments come into sharp contrast. On the one hand, the traditionalists cite holy writ as absolutely prohibiting the practice as an abomination in the eyes of God (Leviticus, Chapter 18, verse 22), and therefore incompatible in one claiming to represent God to the people. On the other, there are those who claim that, within a loving relationship, it is as much a human facsimile of the love of God as similar acts within a loving heterosexual relationship. The first group claims that respect can only be granted within certain absolute unalterable parameters that have been laid down by the law of God or man. The second group implies that the very existence of a person involves rights that cannot be overridden or circumscribed without very strong reasons (e.g. because they conflict with another's rights). Two different aspects of the problem are becoming confused here. Whether or not I personally respect A is as much a matter of my beliefs and attitudes as of his. Whether or not I personally respect a person who engages in self-damaging behaviour by smoking, should he nevertheless be accorded the general respect of the community. It could be argued, for example, that he should have designated areas on public transport where he can smoke if he wishes. However, although it may be in the parents' interest that their beliefs be respected, even if they are harmful to themselves, their interests and those of the child may not coincide.

Savulescu and Momeyer suggest that the rationality of the belief is important, in that irrational belief interferes with a person's ability to exercise autonomy, and is not in his or her interest.[16] This begs the question of what constitutes irrational belief. Some would argue that any religious belief, since it is not amenable to scientific examination, is irrational. They argue that although the choices on which an autonomous decision is made need not be rational, the beliefs on which it is based must be. Thus, for example, if a person decides to continue smoking while knowing that it has a high chance of damaging his health, because he finds smoking pleasant, then that is an autonomous decision based a rational belief. However, if despite knowing and understanding all of the health risks, he decides to continue smoking because he believes it will improve his health, then this is an irrational belief, and the decision is therefore not truly autonomous. Savulescu and Momeyer relate this to the need to respect the refusal of Jehovah's Witnesses to accept blood transfusion. They point out that since Jehovah's Witnesses believe that if they refuse blood and die as a result, they will attain eternal bliss, but if they accept the blood, even if they live, they will turn to dust when they do eventually die, it is rational to choose eternal bliss and refuse blood. However, they try to make a case that the very belief in the universal embargo on accepting any blood by any route is irrational by the very terms of the Jehovah's Witnesses' own belief system, since Jesus himself advocated the drinking of his blood in instituting the Eucharist. They suggest therefore that where a belief can be shown to be internally irrational, it behoves the doctor to attempt to educate the patient out of this irrationality, by bringing to their notice the facts which make the belief irrational. However, they weaken their case by stating that 'respect for autonomy is not the only ground for non-intervention in another person's life. It is surely enough that it is his life, and that he ought to be allowed to do what . . . he chooses'.[16] They seem to be saying that irrational beliefs should be contested, but in the end respected, even if they interfere with the proper exercise of autonomy. That this is not adhered to in practice is demonstrated by a recent court case in which leave was granted to a hospital authority to withdraw artificial ventilation from a baby with type 1 spinal muscular atrophy, despite the fact that the parents argued that, as orthodox Jews, not to preserve life was deeply offensive to their religious beliefs.[17] In a comment on the case, a spokesman for the Royal College of Paediatrics and Child Health said that 'this case appears to fit into the "no chance" situation'.[18] That is to say, it is treatment that may delay death but which does not relieve suffering. It is not clear what caused the suffering of the child, other than the discomfort of ventilation, which was already being tolerated. Any suffering would be on the part of the parents in having to live with the knowledge that their child had a fatal condition and this was certainly not relieved by the decision to stop the ventilation – it was made worse. In the reports much is made of the fact that the child was 16 months old, even though most children with this condition are dead by 12 months. It is difficult to see the relevance of this, since to accept that once a person has exceeded their allotted span, be that 1 year or 70 years, it is morally permissible to kill him, is surely untenable.

The *Shorter Oxford Dictionary* gives one definition of respect which I feel comes close to covering this problem of accepting a decision, even if that decision is based on an irrational belief. The definition is 'to treat with consideration; to refrain from interfering with; to spare'.[19] Be that as it may, actions based on religious belief can be rational in Savulescu and Momeyer's terms since if, for example, one believes that adherence to the Law will bring the advent of the Messiah with its attendant blessing to all mankind, to make this one's primary interest is rational.

Should parents therefore have a right and interest in having their beliefs respected to the extent that the State and the local authority should make special health and educational provision for disabled children within their community in order not to offend those beliefs? For Hasidic parents, for example, adherence to the Law of God as interpreted by the Rebbe of their particular sect is not only their prime interest, but it could be seen as their only interest, since if their compliance is complete, all else will follow. Therefore anything which puts an obstacle in the way of following this belief is not in their interest. Since their child is as much under the Law as they are themselves, this applies to the child, too. Any part of the treatment which creates such an obstacle would therefore not be in the child's interest. Whether or not the parents' beliefs need to be respected, do they nevertheless need to be taken into account in the management of the child? On the question of educational provision, the position of special religiously based schools within the UK education system is clear. The 1944 Education Act regularised the position of Anglican schools within state education, establishing religion as an educational need.[20] The Act also gives parents the right to send their children to independent schools provided that these schools offer efficient education. Since the passage of the Education Reform Act 1988,[21] such efficiency is more easily defined in that there is a requirement that children satisfy the assessments of their performance on standard tests of core curriculum subjects. The 1944 Act also requires that all independent schools be subject to inspection, and for a school which has failed such an inspection to continue is a criminal offence. How then does this affect the response to the requirement of a community that their religious beliefs override all other considerations in the provision of education to their children? Is the State required to respect this and act on it? There are two elements to this issue. First, should the children be allowed to attend the religious schools? Secondly, should the State contribute to their education in these schools by providing specialist input to those children who have special needs? The religious community could comply with the spirit of the law by demonstrating that the secular education that is available to the children in their schools compares favourably with national standards. To take another example, namely the apparent difference between Sikhs and Rastafarians with regard to the matter of wearing crash helmets,[22] it seems to be that the Sikhs comply with the spirit of the law in wearing a form of head protection (the turban), whereas the Rastafarians do not. However, this would not solve the problem of provision of special needs resources to the religious schools. A different minority group in a similar position is that of parents who choose to send their children to independent secular schools, who are also not entitled to special needs provision in the school of their choice. Is there any difference between parents who believe that their children get a better deal by going to an independent private secular school, and those who believe that the best deal for their children is to go to an independent private religious school? The educational standards in the private secular schools are usually high, so that they comply with the law. For both groups the special needs provision would be available if their children attended state schools. However, even this is not clear-cut. In a judgement based on the psychological damage done to a Hasidic child required under the terms of his Statement to attend a secular special school,[23] it was ruled that the education authority was required to name a private religious school in the Statement and to pay the cost of special needs provision, on the grounds that the parents had made appropriate provision by placing him in the school. It therefore appears that by requiring that their children, whatever their special needs, have an overriding special need to attend specific religious schools, and to have their other special needs met by the community, the religious communities are supported by the law of the land. In that it relates to the provision of specifically religious needs, this probably does not apply to children in private secular schools. However, in order to comply with the spirit of the law, maintenance of the standards required by the various Education Acts cited should be a duty that they should be required and prepared to accept.

In summary, parents have a right, since it is in their interest, to participate in decisions that affect the education or medical welfare of their children. This involves others in respecting the beliefs of the parents, and the effect that these beliefs have on the decisions that are made, provided that no actual harm accrues to others as a result of the beliefs that are held. However, this does carry with it a duty on the parents to accept any consequences of this – for example, that in all other respects the law is complied with.

References

1 Vandeveer D (1981) Experimentation on children and proxy consent. *J Med Phil.* **6**: 281–93.

2 McCormick RS (1974) Proxy consent in the experimentation situation. *Perspect Biol Med.* **18**: 2–20.

3 Sykes JB (ed.) (1976) *The Concise Oxford Dictionary* (6e). Oxford University Press, Oxford.

4 Simpson JAD and Weiner ESC (eds) (1989) *The Oxford English Dictionary* (2e). Clarendon Press, Oxford.

5 O'Neil R (1983) Determining proxy consent. *J Med Phil.* **8**: 389–403.

6 In re Eichner, 102 Misc. 2d 184, Ct of App., 52 NY. 2d 263,420 ME. 2d 64, 436 N.Y.S. 2d 266 (1981).

7 *The California Natural Deaths Act* (AB 3060 September 1976).

8 In re Quinlan, 70 NJ 10, 355 A. 2d 647 (1976).

9 Higgs R (1985) A father says 'Don't tell my son the truth.' *J Med Ethics.* **11**: 153–8.

10 Knott L (1996) Fcmale circumcision in Britain. *Matern Child Health.* **21**: 127–9.

11 Abu-Sahlieh SAA (1994) To mutilate in the name of Jehovah or Allah: legitimization of male and female circumcision. *Med Law.* **13**: 575–622.

12 Carlton Television (1999) *Changing Faces.* 24 November.

13 Jones RB (1999) Parental consent to publicity. *J Med Ethics.* **25**: 379–81.

14 Jones RB (2000) Point of view: parental consent to cosmetic facial surgery in Down's syndrome. *J Med Ethics.* **26**: 101–2.

15 Bradney A (1993) *Religions, Rights and Laws.* Leicester University Press, Leicester, p. 4.

16 Savulescu J and Momeyer RW (1997) Should informed consent be based on rational beliefs? *J Med Ethics.* **23**: 282–8.

17 Dyer C (1997) British court allows terminally ill baby to die. *BMJ.* **315**: 1398.

18 Cresswell J (1997) Treatment denial in line with guidance. *Hosp Doctor.* **4 December**: 9.

19 Brown L (ed.) (1993) *New Shorter Oxford English Dictionary.* Oxford University Press, Oxford.

20 *Education Act 1944.* HMSO, London.

21 *Education Reform Act 1988* HMSO, London.

22 *Motor-Cycle Crash Helmets (Religious Exemptions) Act 1976.* C62. HMSO, London.

23 Regina v Inner London Education Authority ex parte F. (Unreported case. Transcript reference CO\365\88.)

Chapter 8

The interests and rights of the physician

An infringement of an interest can amount to an infringement of a right if 'all other things being equal, an aspect of . . . well-being (his interest) is sufficient for holding some other person(s) to be under a duty'.[1] Therefore the interests and rights of the physician will be considered.

Treatment is a contract between the patient and the physician in which the interests of both must be considered. Acceding to the request of patients (or the parents of patients) for their beliefs to be respected may result in treatment that not only deviates from the orthodox, but which is also bad practice. To put respect for the autonomy of the patient above respect for the beliefs of the physician, requiring him to collude with what he considers to be bad or unethical practice, is an unacceptable infringement of his interests. It is this requirement to collude that is the heart of the problem, even if it does not actually affect treatment.

What conforms to ethical and proper management of the patient is not straightforward, since it will inevitably involve consideration of what is in the best interest of the patient. On the other hand, colluding with ineffective or damaging treatment is in the best interest of neither the physician nor the patient. For the physician, harm could accrue from the opprobrium that such practice would receive from colleagues, and the potential for litigation from the patient. For the patient, harm could obviously accrue from the adverse outcome of poor treatment.

Gillon[2] argues that the physician should not be required to collude with giving what he considers to be inadequate treatment, since not only is it a duty of a doctor to do no harm, but also to provide the best care possible is a supererogatory duty that other professions do not have. This is different from the obligation that, say, a shopkeeper has to his customers, or an airline pilot has to transport his passengers safely, in that the doctor has an obligation to dissuade his patients from a course of treatment which they may want, but which he feels is potentially harmful to them. The doctor may also have a duty to see that the best is done for all of his patients by ensuring an equitable distribution of resources, and so far as possible ensuring that those resources are adequate. It may be that, as a private citizen rather than as a doctor, he also has a duty to see that resources are distributed equitably to the whole community, and not to do anything which would upset that distribution.

One definition of an interest is that which, if infringed, causes harm. If it is in the interest of the physician that his treatment is ethical and effective, what harm is caused to the physician if he fails to fulfil this obligation? Apart from the fact that it will lessen his own satisfaction, it can be argued that a physician is only able to fulfil his role if he has the trust of his patients, his colleagues and the public. It is therefore in his interest to fulfil his obligations both for his personal satisfaction and to enable him to continue in practice with the good will of patients and colleagues.

Sevensky views the doctor–patient relationship as a covenant akin to that between God and mankind. This he claims is preferable to relying on codes and contracts in that it emphasises the care worker's indebtedness to society and to God, the obligations of the patient as a covenant partner, and the 'faithfulness and trust necessitated by the patient's vulnerability'.[3] The doctor–patient relationship is a shared responsibility, but this in no way diminishes the demand for technical proficiency.

Does claiming a right impose a duty on the claimant? Is the duty to fulfil one's obligations, for example, so tied up with claiming the right to practise that it is part of the physician's interests? Emson[4] is quite clear that claiming a right imposes corresponding duties on the recipient of that right.[4] If the rights of an individual derive from that individual's autonomy, then the rights of all members of the community can only be preserved by voluntary limitation of individual autonomy. For example, if a man who is infected with HIV claims the right to confidentiality, that imposes a duty of disclosure on him to protect the rights of his partner. For a physician, claiming the right to practise imposes a duty to provide good care. To what extent, therefore, is there an obligation to accept a duty when claiming a right, and to what extent should this obligation be enforced? Lesser suggests that such obligations do not necessarily require consent from the person with the duty if there is an adequate reciprocal obligation. For example, 'since no rich person can know for certain that they will not one day be destitute, to impose . . . an obligation on the rich to help the poor is not in fact to impose an obligation that is unilateral in principle, although it may be so in practice'.[5] Secondly, consent is not required if there is an already existing moral obligation to act in that way, re-inforcing the idea that a physician does have such a duty to comply with his obligations in his own interest.

Gordon looks at the justification within the Jewish tradition for respecting patient autonomy, and he contrasts this with more rigid interpretations of Halakhah 'which disregard the intimacy of the doctor–patient relationship'.[6] He makes much of the need for the doctor's relationship with the patient to be compassionate, and he quotes an old rabbi of his childhood: 'Kinderlech, az ihr hobt kein rachmones, far wos seid ihr Yiden? (Children, if you have no compassion, what makes you Jews?)'. This he transforms into 'doctors, if you have no compassion, what makes you doctors?'.[6] However, one can have compassion for a patient without agreeing to everything that he asks. It may be more compassionate to deny his requests, in the interest of both patient and physician. Wilson claims that, provided the patient has not given the doctor a specific mandate to decide for him, what the patient wants should always prevail even if it is manifestly not in his best interest, the function of the doctor being to find out the patient's wants.[7] He does not address the dilemma of the doctor who is faced with patient wishes that are opposed to his own ethical values. Neither Gordon nor Wilson address the patient's duty of compassion to the doctor – compassion is a two-way process. To paint the doctor into a corner where he has no way out but to deny his own conscience is not compassionate, and is certainly not in the physician's interest.

Harris asks whether doctors qua doctors have an obligation to treat patients and to save lives that transcends the obligation that we all have to come to the aid of our distressed fellows, and he concludes that they do not.[8] However, because of their special expertise, doctors are more often placed in the situation of being able to save lives than are others. He cites two cases, one of a diabetic in a hypoglycaemic coma, and the other of a patient who is dying as a result of massive blood loss. He claims that if the doctor does not give glucose to the first patient or replacement blood to the second, knowing that they will die if they are not treated but will live if they are treated, then he is responsible for their deaths, and could come to harm if he was deemed so responsible. However, such patients do not die of lack of treatment – they die of lack of glucose or lack of blood. If, for example, the blood loss resulted from an attack, the failure to treat would not absolve the attacker from a charge of murder. Harris suggests that because a doctor is specially trained to save life, although he is under no more obligation than anyone else to use his skills, we judge him more harshly if he does not do so.[8] Davis points out that it is one thing for a doctor not to respond to a call for help at, say, the scene of a road accident, but quite another for him not to comply with an undertaking entered into by accepting a particular job or a particular patient.[9] Although the doctor in the above examples is not responsible for the deaths of the two patients, he cannot be absolved from moral responsibility, since he not only had it in his power to save them, but he had undertaken to do so. Although what constitutes proper treatment may be arguable, the obligation to treat is not, once the responsibility has been accepted. On this basis it would be the physician's duty, and therefore in his best interest, to treat a patient who was accepted in his practice, but not necessarily one who was encountered casually.

What is it to accept an obligation or a duty? Schumaker describes three uses of the word 'duty'.[10] The first relates to the Stoics' concept of officia, that it is one's duty to do what is most appropriate in the circumstances. This leads to a circular argument – I ought to do something it is my duty to do, and it is my duty to do something that I ought to do. Of more relevance is the second use of the word – that we discharge our duty if we fulfil our responsibilities. On this basis it could be said that as a citizen we have a duty to obey laws which are not manifestly unjust. However, we are not absolutely bound to fulfil that duty if it conflicts with another duty. Schumaker cites the physician's duty to devote long hours to his practice, versus his duty as a husband and father to devote time to his family – the conflict between the interests of his family and those of his patients influencing his idea of what is in his own best interest. The third concept of duty is a negative one which demands that no wrong is done. Provided that one adheres to the minimum standards required, duty has been done. Schumaker then introduces the concept of covenant, in which what binds us to our fellows is based on what we have received from them and on common tradition. 'Contracts are made and discharged for mutual advantage. Covenants are based upon obligations generated by past relationships and have "a gratuitous, growing edge" which continually creates future relationships.'[10] The idea of a covenant generates not just a duty to conform to the norms and laws of the wider community, but an obligation to do so which goes beyond the strict requirements of the law.

It is in the physician's interest to comply with the legal and ethical requirements of practice. This would include, for example, obtaining the patient's informed consent to treatment. Although the patient need not be compliant, it is in the physician's interest that once a treatment plan has been agreed, and informed consent has been given to it, that the patient accepts an obligation to either comply with the treatment, or inform the physician if he or she is not doing so.

Although it is accepted that the doctor has duties and the patient has rights, there is less acceptance that the reverse is true although, as Meyer points out, the idea is not new.[11] In 1847, the American Medical Association published a code of medical ethics that contained a long list of patient duties. These ranged from the duty to choose qualified physicians, to following the advice given and even being eternally grateful for the cure afterwards. There is no mention anywhere in this code of patient rights. In that the patient now has the right to make autonomous decisions about the choice of physician, and the subsequent course that the treatment takes, Meyer claims that a tacit partnership exists between patient and physician, and that such a partnership implies duties on both sides, as well as rights. He lists a series of duties. The first duty, to communicate openly, can be seen as the direct counterpart of the doctor's duty to inform the patient. This includes 'a duty to be honest about why the patient seeks the healthcare professional's assistance; a duty to give as good a medical history as possible; a duty . . . to tell the healthcare professional whether they are following previously agreed procedures (and if not, offer some explanation, for instance report on the side-effects of a drug). This duty goes beyond the obligation to avoid lying. It includes a duty to avoid withholding information believed to be relevant, because this may ultimately affect the patient's participation in treatment.'[11] This he feels includes a duty 'to . . . see nurses and doctors for what they are, skilled and concerned professionals with limited powers'.[11] This he claims is a duty which goes to the heart of the patient's role in collaborative decision making, since the assessment of the healthcare professional's abilities clarifies the patient's role in his own healthcare. Accepting these duties is not an ideal behaviour of the perfect or virtuous patient, but a moral obligation for all autonomous patients and thus in the interest of the physician. If it is accepted that they have a duty to their advisers by the act of seeking their advice, then that duty must involve an openness about whether or not to accept that advice and a willingness to do everything in their power to comply with it once they have accepted it.

Holm discusses this in the context of the non-compliant patient.[12] Provided that the patient can make an autonomous decision, she has no requirement to comply with treatment. However, entering into a covenant with the doctor implies a duty to comply with the recommendations of that doctor in exchange for the right to treatment. If the patient is expected to make an autonomous evaluation of the treatment once he or she has been given all of the facts, then 'compliance' is the wrong word since it implies that doctor knows best and the patient's opinions are of no interest. Holm makes the point that patients with chronic disease rapidly become expert on the way in which the disease affects them, so that even though the doctor may know more about the disease in general, the patients should be allowed to control treatment in themselves. He cites as examples the epileptic or diabetic who modifies the regime prescribed in order to lead a more acceptable life, free from side-effects, even though this may result in suboptimal control. In other words, the doctor and the patient should be partners – not one the compliant, obedient patient and the other an all-powerful doctor. This mutually dependent relationship fits Schumacher's idea of a covenant. Holm goes further in claiming that 'it is not patients who should comply with their doctors' demands, but doctors who should comply with their patients' informed and considered desires'.[12] However, are patients' informed and considered desires necessarily either in their own interest or within the physician's ability to comply without compromising his own professional integrity?

If it is accepted that patients have obligations if the physician's interests are not to be infringed, can these be enforced without their consent? And if so, how should they be enforced? Benjamin sees two main areas of patient obligation, namely full and complete disclosure of all relevant information, and co-operation in mutually agreed treatment plans.[13] Failure on the part of the patient to fulfil these obligations infringes the physician's interest by depriving them of the right to 'fulfil the standards of excellence of their . . . practices. . . . When lay participants have different ends or goals and withhold these from the physician the integrity of the practice as a whole is undermined.'[13] Benjamin cites as an example the case of a man about to undergo triple-bypass surgery with the objective, as expressed by him to a psychiatrist, of ending a burdensome life by submitting to the operation and dying as a result. Since the man had forbidden the psychiatrist to tell the surgeons of this, the problem is superficially one of the duties of the psychiatrist to the patient, the surgeons and the patient's family. However, it also concerns the patient's duty to the surgeons, since 'by withholding certain information, he appears to be manipulating them into serving as agents of his death'.[13] He claims that 'if the patient has an ethical obligation to provide this information to the surgeons, the psychiatrist . . . has strong grounds for persuading him to release her from her pledge of confidentiality, and if this fails, for going directly to the surgeons',[13] thus claiming that the patient's duty to the surgeons justifies overriding his autonomous decision not to disclose the information, and breaking the psychiatrist's promise not to do so.

The main difficulty lies in knowing how to define the relationship between the physician and the patient. Ladd suggests that this is akin to Aristotelian friendship.[14] However, Ketchum and Pierce point out that the patient and the physician are not equals, since patients are private individuals whereas physicians have a political power base in the institutions which govern and control their practice.[15] They therefore claim that this cannot be Aristotle's perfect friendship between equals, but rather it is that between father and son, or between ruler and ruled. Given this inequality, they claim that this puts additional obligations on the physician, and they imply that for the patient the significance of the rights within the relationship is greater than any duties they may have.

However, of the types of friendship described by Aristotle,[16] the one which most closely describes the doctor–patient relationship is friendship based on utility. This occurs between opposites, 'because each, being eager to secure what he happens to lack himself, is prepared to give something else in return'.[16] He cites as examples rich and poor, or scholar and ignoramus. In the context of the doctor–patient relationship, this would be between one individual with specialised knowledge and one without. He claims that the better person in the friendship – the one with more knowledge, skill or wealth – must be more loved than the other, 'for when the affection is proportionate to merit the result is a kind of equality, which is of course considered to be characteristic of friendship'.[16] This would fit in well with the duties described by the American Medical Association. It is of interest that Aristotle claims that it is only in friendship based on utility that complaints arise, 'because since each associates with the other for his own benefit, they are always wanting the better of the bargain, and thinking that they have less than they should'.[16]

I am not advocating either that the interests of the physician demand compliance from the patient, or that it is never in the interest of the physician to collude with the patient. Two different forms of collusion must be differentiated – first, modifying the treatment to take into account the patient's beliefs, even if they conflict with orthodox treatment (although not to the extent of rendering the treatment inadequate), and secondly, agreeing to co-operate with the patient even though this compromises the adequacy of the treatment. A further problem in discussing collusion is that the patients referred to are children, and decisions are often being taken for them by adults, the parents, the healthcare professionals or even the courts. Like so much else, therefore, the problem of collusion occurs at second hand. In colluding with what may be inadequate treatment, the collusion is not with the opinions and desires of the patient, but with those of their carers. Kearney addresses this problem in relation to the treatment of leukaemia in the children of Jehovah's Witnesses, which is complicated by the refusal of these families to accept blood transfusion.[17] So rigid is this prohibition that if a court order is obtained to give the transfusion, it could result in family disruption and the rejection of the child, although this has never been recorded.[18] Kearney points out that not only are the family's requirements rigid, but also the doctor's often are as well, since the pattern of treatment is often dictated by a strict protocol. In analysing this, he uses De Mause's three possible reactions of an adult to a child in need, namely projective, reversal or empathic reactions. In the projective model, the child serves only as a vehicle for the adult's inner fears, hopes and beliefs. Decisions are based on the needs of the treatment rather than the needs of the child. In reversal, not only is the leukaemia considered separately from the child, but also the decisions are now taken in the best interest of the physician rather than of the child. Kearney cites medico-legal reasons, peer pressure and research needs as the causes of this reversal. He sees this as similar to but less dangerous than the projective model, since the beliefs tend to be less rigid and more susceptible to conversion to an empathic approach in which the total interests of the child are advanced. In the cases that he describes, remission was induced without the use of blood transfusion, which although less likely to ensure success, did ensure that in the long term family disruption did not occur. In taking this empathic approach, again what could have been seen as collusion with less than optimal short-term treatment was in fact good long-term management. It can thus be said to be in the interest of the patient, the parents and the physician.

To what extent therefore do the interests of the patient demand that the physician has a duty to compromise his or her own beliefs so as not to infringe the interest of the patient? Bilu and Witztum addressed the case of an ultra-orthodox Jewish man with severe depressive psychosis.[19] The therapists felt that this was related to internalised guilt about having neglected his father at the time of his death, and they suggested ways of appeasing the father, none of which were effective. The patient explained his behaviour as adherence to the commands of a visiting angel. Attempts to counter the angel's demands with religious arguments also failed, so in association with a Rabbi, a Jewish court consisting of the patient, the therapist and the Rabbi was convened. The patient was allowed to use a ritual of candles and geometric shapes to summon the angel, which was then exorcised, with considerable improvement of the patient as a result.

Was this type of treatment modification actually collusion in the first meaning described above, or more an adjustment to the patient's mind-set, using his own concepts of disease to help his cure? In that it does involve the therapist in collaborating in rituals which he believes to be nonsense, there was an element of collusion of the first kind. The equivalent might be a doctor agreeing to a patient's request that his condition be treated with homeopathy. If the doctor himself believes that homeopathy is an effective method of treatment, then the question of collusion does not occur. However, if he believes it to be useless, and furthermore that more orthodox therapy, for example, with an antibiotic, would be effective, then to agree to the patient's demands is dishonest and constitutes collusion. I think this is equivalent to more than using a placebo, since it lends support to a whole belief system which the doctor believes to be false. It is this element of dishonesty which lies at the heart of collusion, particularly if, as in this situation, it results in treatment which is at best of no value, and at worst harmful.

So-called alternative systems of medicine, such as homeopathy, have much in common with religious belief because they are based not on reproducible scientific evidence, but on the basic attributes of a religion, dogma, paradox, 'ritual and mystery'. If one takes homeopathy as an example, then the initial dogma lies in the very name – homeopathy, meaning 'like cures like', often expressed, as if to emphasise its dogmatic nature, in Latin, *similia similibus curentur*.[20] If you have a headache, then take something to cure it that would give you a headache if you did not have one. There is no evidence for this statement, and in fact the whole concept defies common sense – it is a paradox which is turned into a dogma. If you do not believe it, then you reject the whole. To help belief, play with the paradox, not just like, but like that has been given potency (an important choice of word) by the application of a second paradoxical dogma – that weakness is strength. The greater the dilution, the greater the potency. Dilution itself is not sufficient to potentiate the mixture. Shaking in a particular, ritualistic way (succussion) for a particular period of time is required for that. However, what type of religion is it that has no mystery? This surely is the 'form energy' – the essence of the original substance which permeates the solution as a result of the ritual shaking even if the dilution is so great that not a single molecule of the solute remains in the solution. Since there seems to be no way of convincing people that these therapies have no scientific basis, even though the majority of users are educated professional people,[21] then they could, for the reasons outlined above, be treated as akin to religion. Adherents of religious beliefs generally feel that they derive benefit from such beliefs, so this might form a basis for the claimed effectiveness of the so-called 'alternative therapies' – for like all religions, therapies such as homeopathy work best for those who believe in them most. As in the case, for example, of belief in the power of prayer, the actual result can always be interpreted positively. If you get what you pray for, that is a direct answer – if you do not, it is God demonstrating that he knows best what you need. Similarly, even if the actual disease is not cured by homeopathy, patients will usually claim that they feel better in themselves. Attempts to make homeopathy scientific by conducting controlled trials have not yet yielded convincing results. A review of clinical trials of homeopathy, although it showed some positive results, found that the majority of the trials were so flawed that no firm conclusions could be drawn.[22] It should not be thought that collusion with therapies such as homeopathy is always harmless, even though proponents of the therapies claim that they cause no harm. Although the so-called potencies themselves are harmless, the delay in obtaining proper treatment may not be. If homeopathy and the like can be accepted as being akin to a religion, it might make it easier to offer medical treatment to the adherents of such alternative therapies since, as with a Jehovah's Witness, the dangers of pursuing their beliefs can be made clear to them, and their informed decision to forego orthodox treatment, or to combine it with the unorthodox, can be defined. Sikora describes the use of various forms of alternative therapy as an adjunct to orthodox cancer treatment, aimed at improving the patient's well-being and thereby possibly improving the response to the cancer.[23] In this respect it is exactly similar to respecting the patient's religious faith, or their psychological attitude to the cancer, without compromising the proper treatment of the disease. Only when the patient wishes to substitute the unorthodox for the orthodox completely does the question of collusion arise. It might be argued that this approach colludes with the patient in that it lends support to a system of belief that the therapist may think is nonsense. However, if this is done in combination with orthodox treatment, and it is made clear to the patient that it is their beliefs that are being respected, rather than it being that the therapist believes that the unorthodox treatment has any physical effect, then no collusion is involved. However, if the therapist remains silent, then it could be said that tacit support is being given. This, I believe, applies equally to the patient's religious beliefs. For example, it has always been my practice to provide the necessary reports for patients to go to Lourdes, while at the same time I make it clear that I personally do not believe in miracles.

A more difficult but related problem is that of dealing with a patient whose beliefs are irrational, and which can only be made rational by colluding with his or her prejudices. Faden and Faden discuss the duties of the physician when faced with a patient who is given all the facts of his or her case, understands them, and therefore can be said to be fully informed, but refuses to believe them.[24] In their case, because of her racial prejudice, the patient persisted in refusing treatment because she was white and her physician was black, for which reason she did not believe him. Faden and Faden discuss to what extent the patient should be allowed to take this stance, given that it was her health that was at risk, and that there was no evidence – other than the irrationality of her decision – to suggest that she was demented or otherwise incompetent. They conclude that informed consent, or for that matter informed dissent, relies on the patient not only being fully informed and understanding the information that is given, but also believing it to be true. Almost as an aside, they comment that when the situation was explained to this patient by a white physician, she believed him and consented to treatment. They do not discuss the problem of the inherent collusion with her racial prejudice that this involved, even though it produced the desired result.

Generally speaking, it is in the physician's interest to comply with the law. Sometimes, however, it may be necessary for them to collude with what they consider to be unethical practice in order to do so. For example, the Abortion Act 1967 allows doctors to opt out, on conscientious grounds, of giving patients advice about induced abortion.[25] Although it is not specifically stated in the Act, it is widely assumed that there is a requirement on such doctors, if they are not to lay themselves open to a charge of negligence, to refer the patient to another doctor who will give the necessary advice. It is difficult to see the difference between complying with the request at first hand or at second hand, presenting the original physician with no choice but to participate against his or her own moral beliefs. To refer on is dishonest, but not to refer on may be illegal. Meyers and Woods take this further when considering the problem that county hospitals in California have in providing any abortion services at all because of the reluctance of physicians to take part in them. These authors insist that any physician who invokes the conscience clause in order to avoid performing abortions should be required to justify his or her refusal in terms at least as stringent as those required for one to be recognised as a conscientious objector to service in the armed forces.[26]

A related problem is that of cases where acceding to the patient's wishes involves the doctor in actually breaking the law. Lowe describes the extreme case of a conscious, fully competent patient on a ventilator who asks for the ventilator to be turned off in the certain knowledge that this will result in his death.[27] She argues that, since the doctor also knows that this will inevitably result in death, turning off the ventilator is an act of commission which is tantamount to murder. She goes further in suggesting that this is not merely a refusal to continue treatment, but 'is effectively a request to be killed, and as such ought by no means to be acceded to simply in the name of the patient's right to refuse treatment'.[27] She claims therefore that since turning off a ventilator is an act of commission, committing the act at the request of the patient is no different to committing it without that permission, and therefore both are murder, and therefore clearly not in the physician's interest.

Kennedy goes some way towards addressing this by claiming that the discussion hangs not on whether an act is omitted or committed, but on the question of the causation of the death. Since the doctor is legally required to comply with a competent patient's demand that treatment cease, then he is legally required to turn off the respirator. Therefore what he does is legal. He further claims that, in so far as the ensuing death is due to the lethality of the underlying disease which medical science can do nothing about, turning off the respirator does not kill the patient – it allows him to die.[28]

In the entire discussion, no distinction is made between what is legal and what is ethical or moral. Since the courts have ordered respirators to be turned off in well-defined circumstances where there was no hope of independent life, it is clearly not illegal to turn them off in these circumstances, in this country, at this time. However, the whole thrust of the argument in favour of, for example, a conscience clause in the Abortion Bill is that there is not universal agreement that all that is legal is necessarily ethical.

It is therefore in the interests of the physician that, having accepted an obligation to treat the patient, the treatment should be effective, orthodox and ethical. It is in the physician's interest to fulfil his or her obligations, and for the patient also to fulfil his or her obligations to the physician and the treatment programme. It is also in the physician's interest to keep the law, so far as this is compatible with other considerations and does not conflict with his or her other interests. It may be possible to modify treatment programmes to accommodate the interests of the patient (e.g. by avoiding blood transfusion), but collusion which results in poor or harmful treatment is never in the physician's interest.

References

1 Raz J (1984) Rights-based moralities. In: J Waldron (ed.) *Theories of Rights.* Oxford University Press, Oxford, pp. 182–200.

2 Gillon R (1986) Do doctors owe a special duty of beneficence to their patients? *J Med Ethics.* **12**: 171–3.

3 Sevensky RL (1983) The religious foundations of healthcare: a conceptual approach. *J Med Ethics.* **9**: 165–9.

4 Emson EH (1992) Rights, duties and responsibilities in health care. *J Appl Phil.* **9**: 3–11.

5 Lesser H (1989) Obligation and consent. *J Med Ethics.* **15**: 195–6.

6 Gordon HH (1983) The doctor–patient relationship. *J Med Phil.* **8**: 243–55.

7 Wilson J (1986) Patients' wants versus patients' interests. *J Med Ethics.* **12**: 127–30.

8 Harris J (1983) Must doctors save their patients? *J Med Ethics.* **9**: 211–18.

9 Davis JA (1983) Commentary. *J Med Ethics.* **9**: 218–19.

10 Schumaker M (1979) Duty. *J Med Ethics.* **5**: 83–5.

11 Meyer MJ (1992) Patients' duties. *J Med Phil.* **17**: 541–55.

12 Holm S (1993) What is wrong with compliance? *J Med Ethics.* **19**: 108–10.

13 Benjamin M (1985) Lay obligations in professional relations. *J Med Phil.* **10**: 85–103.

14 Ladd J (1979) Legalism and medical ethics. *J Med Phil.* **4**: 70–80.

15 Ketchum SA and Pierce C (1981) Rights and responsibilities. *J Med Phil.* **6**: 271–80.

16 Aristotle (1976) *Ethics* (trans. JAK Thomson). Penguin, Harmondsworth, pp. 270, 272, 282.

17 Kearney PJ (1978) Leukaemia in children of Jehovah's Witnesses: issues and priorities in a conflict of care. *J Med Ethics.* **4**: 32–5.

18 Great Ormond Street Hospital for Children NHS Trust (1996) *Child Protection Policies: procedures and guidance.* Great Ormond Street Hospital for Children NHS Trust, London, p. 125.

19 Bilu Y and Witztum E (1994) Culturally sensitive therapy with ultra-orthodox patients: the strategic employment of religious idioms of distress. *Isr J Psychiatry Rel Sci.* **31**: 170–82.

20 Bayley C (1992) Homeopathy. *J Med Phil.* **18**: 129–43.

21 Clouser KD and Hufford DJ (1993) Non-orthodox healing systems and their knowledge claims. *J Med Phil.* **18**: 101–6.

22 Kleijnen J, Knipschild P and Gerben TR (1991) Clinical trials of homeopathy. *BMJ.* **302**: 316–23.

23 Sikora K (1998) *Eureka.* BBC Radio Four, 8 March.

24 Faden R and Faden A (1977) False belief and refusal of medical treatment. *J Med Ethics.* **3**: 133–6.

25 *The Abortion Act 1967.* HMSO, London.

26 Meyers C and Woods RD (1996) An obligation to provide abortion services: what happens when physicians refuse. *J Med Ethics.* **22**: 115–20.

27 Lowe SL (1997) The right to refuse treatment is not a right to be killed. *J Med Ethics.* **23**: 154–8.

28 Kennedy I (1997) Commentary 3: a response to Lowe. *J Med Ethics.* **23**: 161–3.

Chapter 9

The interests and rights of minority groups

Most of the discussion so far has been about the individual. What are the individual's interests, needs, rights and responsibilities? Yet when dealing with the problems of treating disabled children within a minority community, it is the identity of the group as a whole that is the overriding influence. The factor that determines what in practice can and cannot be done, and what is and is not acceptable, is the group's concept of itself and what is needed to maintain its own integrity. For example, all of the children within the Hasidic community, disabled or able-bodied, attend schools that are run and maintained by the community. However, even within the community there are a number of different sects, each owing allegiance to its own Rebbe, and each with its own religious practice. This results in sects running their own schools to which children of other sects are not sent. In an article purporting to be a conversation between the headmaster of one of these sectarian schools and his daughter,[1] the latter asked why the local education authority Roman Catholic school was so new and bright and clean, compared with their old broken-down schmaterlich (messy, unkempt) building. The headmaster explained to her that the local education authority cares for Christians and supports their schools, but does not care for Jews, and that 'this is called anti-Semitism'.[1] What he did not say was that there are two Jewish schools maintained by the same local education authority – one orthodox and the other reform, but neither conforming to the tenets of his sect. The existence of these mutually exclusive sectarian schools has practical consequences. For example, one way to enable the Hasidic children to receive therapy within their own community, without putting too great a burden on the services available, would be to resource one school to which all of the disabled children would be sent. However, this idea did not get off the ground because of the refusal of the parents of one sect to send their children to a school run by another sect.

There are two main questions here. First, do minority groups, within and possibly at odds with the main culture, have interests and rights as a group different from and additional to the main culture, and in addition to the interests and rights of individual members of the group? Secondly, if they do, how are we to determine in general which groups have these rights? For example, the claim that is implicit in the above article,[1] that the local authority was being anti-Semitic by funding schools for some Jewish sects but not others, could only be justified if all subgroups were entitled to equal rights. Two factors which might influence whether a subgroup has specific rights assigned to it alone are the length of time for which it has been established, and how large it is. Can it be 50 people, or ten, or even just one person? Can it be a subgroup within a minority group?

There are problems in defining a minority group, even before the question of whether specific rights should be assigned to it is discussed. For example, Corvino asks 'how much African-American blood must a person have to be African-American?'.[2] Packer defines a minority as 'a group of people who freely associate for an established purpose where their shared desire differs from that expressed by the majority rule'.[3] He emphasises that it is a free association, which is exemplified by the adult Hasids, since they are free to leave at any time. However, this cannot be clearly asserted for children of any group, since they may not be competent to choose. Even for adults it is not clear that they have an unfettered right to withdraw, since their upbringing and education, concentrating as they do on religious studies at the expense of secular qualifications, do not give them the tools to enable them to cope in a secular society.

Packer defines two types of minority. The positive associate to share a common life plan that is different from that of the majority, and the negative associate to defend themselves against discriminatory behaviour, although for Jews during pogroms and the Holocaust the two merged. Association on the grounds of religion is cultural association, and Packer quotes Kymlica, stating that 'membership in a culture is qualitatively different from membership in other associations, since our language and culture provide the context within which we make our choices',[3] concluding that special rights are justified to maintain cultural integrity. As Packer points out, this view supports group rights against the rights of members of the group in order to maintain such integrity, and justifies restricting freedom to leave the group. However, he also points out that cultures are not static, and that attempts to make them so by restricting freedom lead to an ossification of restrictive practices. He quotes Nino: 'a liberal cannot value all these relations (with other members of his community) so much that he values their forcible imposition'.[3] Although groups such as the Hasidim would not see their way of life as being forced on them, they would encourage such 'ossification', since the Law of God is static in that it is eternal. Packer attempts to balance what are actual needs against available resources if fulfilling minority rights involves for example, a disproportionate distribution of resources, by the formula 'expressed desires + genuine needs against real possibilities',[3] which enables such conflicting claims to be compared and set against the available resources. The International Covenant on Civil and Political Rights states that religious groups should not be denied the right 'to enjoy their own culture', but there is no requirement on Government to help them to do so.[3] Packer sums up as follows: 'the content of minority rights is in the protection . . . guaranteed to persons belonging to minorities for the pursuit of their ideals and plans . . . which do not require uniformity; where uniformity is required . . . and in establishing priorities, the majority rule applies'.[3]

Can one have a wider definition of a minority, based on a claim to rights? Cooper defines such a group 'as any group within a multi-cultural state which claims for itself group rights . . . such that bare membership of the group entitles one to the right'.[4] He claims that in Canada the rights of the minority native culture versus the European Canadian culture, and of the minority francophone culture versus the anglophone culture, require a consensus which harmonises the common ground in the two cultures, each enriching the other without sidelining either. Thus the 'three pathologies', 'the extinction . . . , the manipulative . . . and the assimilation syndromes, through which, by one means or another, the dominant majority culture replaces the minority culture, can be avoided'.[4] He talks of the 'terminus of history . . . being a world community of . . . people who agree in their fundamental beliefs about the way the world is'.[4] This is quite unrealistic when dealing with religious minorities such as the Hasidim. It is precisely because they do not agree with the majority culture about the way the world is that the problem arises, since they see their interests as being best served by obedience to the Law of God, which precludes any compromise or consensus.

Raikka claims that theories of justice are based on the moral intuitions that we have obligations to minority protection.[5] She asks 'Can theories of justice be falsified simply by showing that they do not match with some of our intuitions? If there is a clear intuition that there are obligations to minority protection, is it stronger than the clear intuition that drives us to think otherwise? Is there a clear intuition that there are obligations to minority protection?.' She claims that such intuitions are not easily defined and are not universally accepted. For example, the claim that movement rights of the majority should be curtailed in order to prevent incursion into minority tribal lands is often hotly disputed. Nevertheless, minority cultures exist within multicultural societies, so some sensitivity to their needs is required. The problem lies in deciding to what extent such sensitivity should be embodied in minority group rights.

One mark of cultural integrity is language. To what extent should this be taken into account when dealing with people in an official capacity? In Wales at the beginning of the twentieth century, speaking Welsh was discouraged, and any child who was found doing so at school would have to wear a board round his or her neck bearing a message such as 'I must not speak Welsh in school'.[6] All teaching was done in English, and all dealings with officialdom were conducted in English. At that time Welsh speakers, although a minority in the UK, were the majority in Wales, but by suppressing the language the English not only maintained their hold on the government of the Principality, but actually for a time made English the language of the Welsh elite. My father, although he was able to understand his Welsh-speaking father, was proud that he himself could not speak Welsh. Similarly, a Flemish colleague told me that when he was a boy, the family spoke French (the language of the educated class) rather than Flemish (the language of the lower uneducated classes). This political value of language is illustrated by Harold Pinter's play *Mountain Language*,[7] in which a conquering power controls a subservient people by forbidding the use of its language. Kymlicka points out that there is a long tradition, going back through Marx and Engels to JS Mill and beyond, that regarded it as a positive blessing for 'an inferior and more backward portion of the human race' such as a Breton or a Welshman to be absorbed by 'highly civilised and cultivated people', even if this meant losing their culture and language in the process.[8] Clearly the claim here is that it is in the interests of the 'backward' culture to be integrated into the more civilised one. Today the situation is changing. For example, Welsh is now one of the official languages of the UK, and all official correspondence originating in the Principality is presented in both languages.

Welsh is a long-established language in the UK, with the exception of a small enclave in Chile it is restricted to the UK, and even then it is geographically circumscribed. However, over the past 50 years the number of linguistic minorities in the UK has risen sharply, all long established in their original countries, but only recently established here. In an inner-city borough with a population of about 150 000, I counted 152 languages used by the patients attending my clinic. Unlike the Welsh, all of whom speak English as well, many of these people speak only their own language. What criterion should be used to decide which of these languages should become official? Should it be that the language is indigenous to the UK? English itself might not fare too well on that one! Should it be the size of the group speaking the language? Could it be said, for example, that the small number of people who speak

Twi have less need to understand what the doctor is saying to them than the large number who speak Bengali? Or should it be the length of time for which the community has been established here? This could in fact be counter-productive, since the long-established communities have had time to learn English, whereas the more recent immigrants have not. It is claimed by some that everyone has the right to have an interpreter present at any official consultation. The financial cost of this would be prohibitive, and would cut other services, but on the other hand the consultation is a complete waste of time if neither side can understand the other.

This question of minority group interests can be related to the problem of minority group schools. It is in the interest of all that children should be taught in an environment which is safe, clean, pleasant and hygienic, by teachers who are competent. However, there might be disagreement as to what constitutes competence. In Wales, for example, it is virtually impossible for a teacher who does not speak Welsh to get a job, even if that job does not involve the use of Welsh. Any group that wishes to educate its children in its own schools has the right to do so, since private schools are legal in this country, but it also has the corresponding duty to comply with standards of, for example, hygiene, health and safety. To be expected to submit to the same system of inspection that applies to all other schools, and to comply with the findings of that inspection, even if it means closing schools, cannot be seen to be anti-minority. It is in the interest of the members of the group – the pupils – and therefore presumably in the interest of the group as a whole. This is cross-cultural and applies to all, and it is difficult to see how it can offend any religious or cultural beliefs or be seen not to be in the interest of the group. However, to insist on adherence to the requirements of legislation controlling what is taught, or the training of teachers, is more controversial because it impinges on religious or cultural beliefs, and could therefore perhaps be seen as directly equivalent to the suppression of a first language. For the Hasidim, for example, true learning consists solely of the study of the religious texts, secular studies being regarded as of little or no value. A learned man in this culture is one who is steeped in the Talmud. For instance, I was told by one Hasidic rabbi that Albert Einstein was not an ornament to world scholarship, but a loss to Talmudic scholarship!

It is pertinent here to consider two types of cultural minority, which are not necessarily mutually exclusive. The first category is that in which the group maintains its own integrity, speaking its own language, practising its own religion, but leaving itself open to aspects of surrounding cultures, and to modification of its own culture by them. As Waldron says, the francophone Québécois loses nothing by eating Chinese food, listening to Italian opera or telling her children German fairy tales.[9] However, we should note, that Kymlicka takes issue with Waldron's contention that this indicates that there is a kaleidoscope of cultures in which such people live, rather than their living in their own culture. He points out that 'this is not moving between societal cultures. Rather it is enjoying the opportunities provided by the diverse societal culture'.[10] The second category is different in that the surrounding culture is seen as inimical to the group's identity. Anything that smacks of assimilation into the host group, or contamination by the host culture, is vigorously resisted. Groups such as the Hasidim belong to this category. All outside influences are often strictly controlled, with little or no exposure to media such as television or cinema, and those secular books that are allowed are mutilated if they are found to contain material that is offensive to the group. For example, non-kosher animals in children's picture books will be cut out to avoid exposing the child to them. Follesdal asks to what extent a 'just state' can allow such restriction on members by cultural minorities, and suggests that 'it seems implausible to hold that all aspects of minority culture should be tolerated in the name of equal respect'.[11] The case is easiest where the restrictions cause actual physical harm to the members, for example, female circumcision, but Follesdal also cites schools in which information about the wider culture is withheld. He makes the point that escape is possible because of the option of exit from the group, but the social consequences of such an exit do not usually make it viable. Furthermore, if the education is restricted, escape from the group is made doubly difficult. Here there would seem to be a conflict of interests not between the minority group and the wider culture, but between the minority group and its own members.

Language again provides a model for these two types of minority culture. If Welsh and Scottish Gaelic are compared, it will be found that Welsh continually incorporates new words, whereas Gaelic seeks an existing word or word combination within the language to serve as a substitute. For example, there was a furore in the Scottish press some years ago because an announcer in a Gaelic radio broadcast had used the word 'spaghetti'. This was seen as signalling the beginning of the end of the purity of the language. It is significant that Welsh is a thriving language, whereas Gaelic remains the language of a diminishing constituency of native speakers and an intellectual cultural elite. Kymlicka claims that 'any language which is not a public language becomes so marginalised that it is likely to survive only amongst a small elite, or in a ritualised form, not as a living and developing language underlying a flourishing culture'.[10]

It may be relevant to consider the effect that the group's origin has on its claim to specific rights. Kymlicka distinguishes between those who have made a conscious decision to move to another country from their original homeland in order, for example, to afford their families greater opportunities, and those who have been forcibly assimilated into the state.[10] He and Walzer, who makes a similar distinction,[12] claim that the former are likely to assimilate more easily into the host culture, as part of that conscious decision, while the latter are likely to resist integration by demanding their own culture, language or territorial integrity, even if this means conflict or even secession. Some commentators imply that the group which has come in order to gain social advantage has a duty to assimilate. To take a rather silly example, during a recent visit of the Pakistan cricket side to the UK, a former Tory cabinet minister claimed that those British citizens whose families had originated in Pakistan, who supported the Pakistan side in the Test matches, were showing great disloyalty to their own country and would never integrate and become fully British.

For groups such as the Hasidim, this division breaks down. Many of them have moved to the UK from their homelands in Eastern Europe, not due to personal desire but as a life-preserving necessity that was forced on them by the brutality of others. They are presumably in the UK because, if they were ever given the choice, they chose to come here rather than, say, the USA. However, the fact that they had to go somewhere is chance not choice, and they remain a minority dispossessed of their 'homeland', the homeland of their Judaism, resisting integration in order to hang on to what remains of this homeland. Their primary loyalty lies with this 'homeland' rather than with the host country. This is perhaps a factor that distinguishes between two types of immigrant – the true refugee (not just the Hasidim), and the so-called economic migrant.

With the Hasidim, who bore the brunt of the Nazi Holocaust, there is an imperative to resist integration lest the destruction of their identity, having failed in the gas chambers, succeeds by this means instead. It is this which perhaps singles out the Jewish community in general and the Hasidim in particular from all other minorities. Throughout Christian history the Jews have been diabolised as the Deicides, the people who put God to death. In fact this is theologically and historically inaccurate, since Christ died because of the sins of all mankind, not just the Jews, and it was the ancestors of modern-day Italians, the Romans, who actually carried out the execution. Had it been the Jews, Jesus would have been stoned to death (Acts, Chapter 8, verses 58–60). However, no pogrom in history has ever come close to the Holocaust in its severity and far-reaching effect on the Jewish community, and in the extent of the debt owed to it not only by those directly involved, the Nazis, but also by the Gentile community as a whole which stood by and did nothing, even turning away shiploads of Jews who had escaped and returning them to persecution.

Because such a debt exists, it must be asked whether the Jewish community has a special case. Is the debt that is owed to them so great that no one has the right to question the way in which they conduct themselves within their own community? Kymlicka claims that 'since many refugees flee their homeland precisely to be able to continue practising their . . . culture, which is being oppressed by the government, . . . [they] arguably should, in principle, be able to re-create their societal culture in some other country if they so desire'.[10] He points out that since their claim is against the persecuting government, it is difficult to know which other country has the duty to service their right.

A partial answer to this question of whether any group can ever be considered to be such a special case that it is exempt from the constraints that apply to all other groups is seen, paradoxically, in Germany, by the response to attempts to discuss the management of severely disabled people, euthanasia and abortion. What is being claimed is not making the Jews a special case because they were persecuted, but making the Germans a special case because they did the persecuting. Singer and Kuhse have had difficulty addressing conferences and student bodies on these subjects in German-speaking countries over the past seven or eight years.[13] Although they claim that their views are misrepresented, and that things which do not represent their views are continually used against them, the argument of their opponents is that by defining a person as a being who is rational and self-conscious, so that some human beings, for example, neonates, are not persons, they are devaluing those human beings and opening the way for them to be denied the rights that are afforded to persons, be they humans or chimpanzees.[13] They claim that by attempting to suppress their views, their opponents are themselves acting like Nazi brown-shirts, breaking up meetings where rational debate was taking place. Their opponents claim that their views lend academic respectability to the concept that some lives are more valuable than others, and justify such behaviour as skinhead attacks on the disabled. Whether or not that is true, in the UK, where no such restriction on freedom of speech is practised, legal decisions restricting the rights of disabled people would be hotly disputed, whereas this is not the case in Germany. Recent decisions have required disabled people in a community home to remain indoors except at specific times, because their behaviour might offend the neighbours, and have also banned disabled people from holiday resorts because their presence would lower the prices that could be charged for holidays.[14] The opponents of Singer and Kuhse quote the Federal Advice and Information Union for Victims of National Socialist Persecution: 'Singer . . . denies human beings the attribute of humanness and therefore makes them available to be killed. We have had experience of that, . . . and not only collectively, but in the experiences of numerous survivors.'[13] This argument can also relate to interference by the Gentile community in the running of Jewish communities, many of the members of which have direct experience of the Holocaust, either personally or through close relatives.

Singer and Kuhse rely in part for their defence of open discussion on Mill's example of the morality of corn dealers: 'An opinion that corn dealers are starvers of the poor, or that private property is robbery, ought to be unmolested when simply circulated through the press, but may justly incur punishment when delivered orally to an excited mob assembled before the house of a corn dealer, or when handed about among the same mob in the form of a placard'.[15] The problem with this is whether at the time Mill was writing there was truly a difference between a newspaper article which needed time to be assimilated, and a placard, the impact of which is immediate – it can be argued that now everything is 'handed out in the form of a placard'. Such has been the explosion in communication that an 'excited mob' has immediate access to almost every utterance of leaders. Thus, for example, when a leader of one faction in Ulster reacts in militaristic terms of no surrender, this is heard by anyone with access to a television set, whatever their level of excitement. It seems to me that the claim that was made by the opponents of Singer and Kuhse – that because of their Nazi history, Germans should not be allowed the freedom to discuss matters of medical ethics, a freedom that is otherwise enjoyed throughout the Western world – cannot be justified, since by stifling one aspect of debate in an attempt to prevent a repetition of past crimes, other injustices against disabled people are allowed to flourish unhindered.

In deciding how this relates to interference with the conduct of their own affairs by minority groups, account must be taken of what is being said. For example, if it is being said that they should send their children to secular schools because, without any evidence being produced, their schools are said to be inadequate or unsafe, then this is manifestly unjust. However, if it is being said that their children are entitled to the same quality of education, teacher competence, access to safe premises and to access special needs provision as other children, and that lesser standards will not be tolerated for them solely because they are from a minority, even if the purveyor of the lesser standards is the group itself, then this cannot be seen as antagonistic to them. The first example could be construed as anti-minority if the judgement is made solely on unsubstantiated grounds, whereas the second, although implying that control of schools is necessary, at least applies it to all schools, religious or secular, private or State aided. However, it does impose duties on both sides – on the minority to ensure that their schools meet acceptable standards, and on the wider community to help them to do this, and to recognise when it has been done, as in the recent recognition of two private Muslim schools for grant-aided status and therefore State financial help now that, following appropriate inspection, they have been found to be of an appropriate educational standard.[16,17]

Does this then make the Jews or the Germans a special case? It can be argued that a considerable debt is owed to the former, and that the wider Gentile community, even if it was not directly involved in the Holocaust, cannot escape that debt. In fact, it could be argued that, far from moulding public opinion inside and outside Germany, Nazism and its attendant anti-Semitism arose from it. Certainly in popular writing of the inter-war years, anti-Semitism was the norm when any mention was made of a Jew in works of fiction. For example, consider the following extract from John Buchan's *The Three Hostages*: 'and then Archie did a very silly thing. He said he was Sir Archibald Roylance and wasn't going to be dictated to by any Jew.'[18]

Today the climate is quite different, so that even to question whether restrictions should be placed on people because of their beliefs is regarded as discriminatory. However, if special case status is accepted, it must be that there is an obligation to ensure that the community does not fall behind with regard to the facilities that are available to it. This may sometimes involve hard decisions which superficially appear to go against the religious freedom of the Hasidim. Making present-day Germans a special case is more dubious. Most of the members of the groups of Jews under discussion have either personal or close family claims on the Holocaust debt. On the other hand, it would be difficult to show that many modern-day Germans have benefited from the past persecution, whether or not they have personal or family connections to the perpetrators of the Holocaust. The only difference between making them responsible, and making the Jews responsible for the death of Jesus, is time – the latter happened much longer ago. The Germans are not a special case, and the protesters are wrong in denying them the right to discuss matters of ethical concern, however repugnant they may find them.

Do minorities have a right to have their culture preserved within a majority culture just because it is their wish that it be preserved? Galenkamp points out that the wish to preserve a culture does not necessarily imply that such a culture exists.[19] This was illustrated when, at the time of a General Election, an attempt was made to establish an English National Party to preserve the English national culture, complete with a national costume that resembled the wardrobe of a third-rate production of the *The Yeoman of the Guard*. Galenkamp suggests that rather than accept the wishes of a community to preserve its culture, an overriding criterion for special minority rights should be an assessment of the needs of the culture to be given special rights to protect it from disadvantage.

If the rights of minorities can be clarified, will this solve the problems of giving adequate treatment and education to disabled children within the minority community? Corvino discusses what is being asked for in claiming minority group interests as rights. For example, does being homosexual confer rights which heterosexuals do not have, a special right, or is it the case that homosexuals should not be denied rights that everyone else enjoys, a general right?[2] This is not straightforward. Since, for example, everyone, homosexual or heterosexual, has the right to marry a member of the opposite gender, it could be said that homosexuals are treated no differently to heterosexuals, and are therefore not discriminated against. To ask that they be allowed to marry a person of the same gender is seemingly to ask for special rights for homosexuals because they are homosexuals. However, heterosexuals are allowed to marry the partner of their choice, but this right is denied to homosexuals, and this, the right to marry the partner of one's choice, is a general right, not a specific one.

Similarly, it could be claimed that since all children have an equal right to special needs provision in local education authority schools, the children of the minority community are not discriminated against if these needs are not met in their own schools, and that to ask that they should be is to ask for a special right for them that is denied to the majority children. Yet it may be that the wrong question is being asked. To ask that special needs be met in a minority school may be construed as a special right. To ask that the minority parents be allowed to specify which school their children attend is to uphold a right that is enjoyed, to some extent at least, by the majority of parents, and which is therefore a general right. If it is possible to redefine all allegedly special rights as general rights by altering the wording of the question that is asked, it could be claimed that there is no such thing as a group specific right, and that the claims that minority groups are making can always be stated as a general right that is available to the majority, but denied to them.

In conclusion, therefore, the whole question of group rights and interests is fraught with difficulties. For example, it does not seem helpful to suggest that facilities to enable children within the minority community to receive special needs provision within their own schools should not be provided, since this would be affording the group a specific right, or that they should be provided because this is a general right, since the way in which such a right is interpreted will to some extent depend on what questions are asked. Similarly, the weight that is put on the need to maintain minority cultures within the more general culture will determine whether group specific rights should be considered at all.

References

1 Wallace W (1988) Why is our school so schmaterlich, Daddy? *Times Educ Suppl.* **5 February**.

2 Corvino JF (1996) How not to argue for gay rights. In: J Raikka (ed.) *Do We Need Minority Rights? Conceptual issues.* Martinus Nijhoff, The Hague, pp. 215–35.

3 Packer J (1996) On the content of minority rights. In: J Raikka (ed.) *Do We Need Minority Rights? Conceptual issues.* Martinus Nijhoff, The Hague, pp. 117–78.

4 Cooper WE (1996) Culture vultures and the re-enchantment of citizenship. In: J Raikka (ed.) *Do We Need Minority Rights? Conceptual issues.* Martinus Nijhoff, The Hague, pp. 21–40.

5 Raikka J (1996) Is a membership-blind model of justice false by definition? In: J Raikka (ed.) *Do We Need Minority Rights? Conceptual issues.* Martinus Nijhoff, The Hague, pp. 3–19.

6 Llewellyn R (1951) *How Green Was My Valley.* Penguin, Harmondsworth, p. 295.

7 Pinter H (1991) Mountain language. In: *Plays Four.* Faber & Faber, London.

8 Kymlicka W (1995) Introduction. In: W Kymlika (ed.) *The Rights of Minority Cultures.* Oxford University Press, Oxford, p. 5.

9 Waldron J (1995) Minority cultures and the cosmopolitan alternative. In: W Kymlika (ed.) *The Rights of Minority Cultures.* Oxford University Press, Oxford.

10 Kymlicka W (1995) *Multicultural Citizenship.* Oxford University Press, Oxford, pp. 78, 85, 98.

11 Follesdal A (1996) Minority rights: a liberal contractualist case. In: J Raikka (ed.) *Do We Need Minority Rights? Conceptual issues.* Martinus Nijhoff, The Hague, pp. 59–83.

12 Walzer M (1995) Pluralism: a political perspective. In: W Kymlika (ed.) *The Rights of Minority Cultures.* Oxford University Press, Oxford.

13 Singer P and Kuhse H (1994) Bioethics and the limits of tolerance. *J Med Phil.* **19**: 129–45.

14 Anon (1998) Ausgrenzung von Behinderten (Excluding the disabled). *Pflege Zeitschrift.* **51**: 176.

15 Mill JS (1960) *On Liberty*. JM Dent, London, p. 14.

16 *Channel Four News*. 9 January 1998.

17 Lepkowska D (1998) Muslims given equality of funding. *Times Educ Suppl.* **4255**: 18.

18 Buchan J (1953, first published 1924) *The Three Hostages*. Penguin, London, p. 187.

19 Galenkamp M (1996) The rationale of minority rights: wishes rather than needs? In: J Raikka (ed.) *Do We Need Minority Rights? Conceptual issues.* Martinus Nijhoff, The Hague, pp. 41–57.

Chapter 10

The interests and rights of the host community

The interests of the host community are not straightforward in that some of the members' interests are defined by the subgroup to which they belong. As a result, they include not only interests that are common to all members, but also specific interests. It is in the interest of all members of the host community that needs are met by a fair distribution of the available resources. Inevitably, since resources are never limitless, it will never be possible to meet all needs, so some hierarchy of need must be defined. A distinction has already been made between course-of-life needs and adventitious needs, failure to meet the former resulting in course-of-life harm, whereas failure to meet the latter resulted only in a adventitious harm. I have extended the original concept not only to include harm as well as need, but also to include non-biological course-of-life needs. If it is accepted that a cultural need (for example, to conform to the Law of God) is a course-of-life need, then it must be met in order to maintain the well-being of the individual concerned. However, for members of the host community who are, for example, atheists this will not be either an adventitious or a course-of-life need.

Is it in the interest of the host community to meet needs which will require unequal and potentially unjust provision? Vlastos[1] cites the case of a man who, having received a death threat from Murder Inc., requires a disproportionately large share of police time to receive the same level of protection as his fellow citizens. Similarly, Salman Rushdie received a death threat from the Muslim community and therefore was afforded considerably more police protection than the average citizen. Childress points out that this will not necessarily be adequate to meet the need, so they may still be murdered.[2] The claim that the special needs of a minority community merit similar special provision depends on whether, like the potential murder victim, they are in that situation of their own volition. It could be said that neither has any choice in the matter.

Daniels offers two meanings for the term 'rights to healthcare' – first, equal access for everyone to what is available, and secondly, a specific level of healthcare to give what is appropriate for each patient's needs, although who defines that need is unclear. If two individuals have the same level of primary goods, but one has simple tastes that can be satisfied by that level, whereas the other's tastes are more demanding, then providing the latter with a greater proportion of goods in order that he may achieve satisfaction cannot be justified, since a 'more modest taste would still service (his) . . . needs'.[3] Tastes are a personal responsibility, not society's responsibility. The same argument can be used with regard to providing for the needs of disabled minority children. In order to receive the same special needs provision as their fellow citizens, they need a disproportionately large share of the time of teachers and therapists, so the majority children will have a smaller share of that resource than would otherwise be the case, since the resource is finite. Vlastos argues that the outcome is just if all children's needs are equally met, to the limits set by the availability of the resource, even if the outcome is less effective than it would otherwise have been. However, if minorities choose to provide schooling which is different from that provided by the State, it could be argued that they should pay for this and for the specialised educational provision required for disabled children.

If it is in the interest of the host community that the interests and rights of members of the community are met, what constitutes these rights? Beauchamp and Childress[4] define rights as justified claims, but this begs two questions. First, who is the claim against? And secondly, who decides what is justified? If a right exists, then some other person or agency has a duty to provide for that right. Unless the holder of the corresponding duty can be identified and made to accept it, then the right is valueless. On the other hand, Wiggins and Derman, albeit discussing needs rather than rights, claim that although a need is 'a legitimate or morally sanctioned demand . . . that has a right to satisfaction, . . . it can make good sense to speak of needs without implying an active obligation on the part of any person to meet these needs'.[5] However, even if a right can be said to exist in the absence of an identified agent with a duty to satisfy that right, in reality it only has value if there is some means of enforcing it.

Lockwood distinguishes between legal and moral or natural rights, and quotes Bentham, stating that 'natural rights . . . is simple nonsense; natural and imprescriptible (i.e. inalienable) rights; rhetorical nonsense – nonsense on stilts'.[6] The plethora of codes of human rights, which set out a series of imprescriptible rights, to which everyone in the world is entitled, and of which they cannot be deprived, bears out Bentham's view, since they are only required because of the inability of the majority of mankind to achieve them. However, one can condemn as morally outrageous people being allowed to starve, for example, without the language of rights.[2] Even with legal rights which circumscribe the entitlement and the responsible implementor of them, there is ambiguity, depending on whether the right obliges someone to do or refrain from doing something. If the right is, for example, special education for a disabled child, then it can be exercised because the agent with the duty can be identified. However, if the right is not being killed without just cause, then although others can be dissuaded from violating that right, and punished if they do violate it, there is no way of restoring it to the original claimant, since he is now dead.

Waldron suggests that if under a moral or legal system a child's interest would be served by assigning a duty to feed him or her, even if no specific agent can be identified as having the duty, the child has a moral or legal right to be fed.[7] However, to claim that a right exists because it ought to, and therefore that the corresponding duty also ought to exist, is a pointless exercise other than to stir the consciences of the well fed.

Shelton claims that the right to healthcare is a moral right, and suggests that a legal right can only exist if 'there exists a . . . duty on the part of ascertainable . . . providers to give medical care to particular persons . . . and the beneficiaries . . . have a legal remedy which they can use to enforce performance of the duty'.[8] Beauchamp and Faden also distinguish between legal and moral rights, and point out that whereas the latter can be used to justify or criticise the former, the reverse is not true. They define rights as 'entitlements a person possesses to some good, service or liberty . . . to be contrasted with privileges, personal ideals, group ideals and acts of charity'.[9] They make a further distinction between negative rights to non-interference, and positive rights to be provided with goods. They illustrate this by differentiating between the right to health (a negative right) and the right to healthcare (a positive right that may contain negative elements involving abstention from action). They claim that 'one person's right entails an obligation on another's part, and all obligations similarly entail rights'.[9]

If it is in an individual's interest to fulfil his or her obligations, then it can be argued that it is also in the interest of the host community. For example, if minority children have a right to care in the religious schools, then this implies that there is an obligation on the host community to provide this care, and thus that it is in its interest to do so. However, Beauchamp and Faden claim that rights are not absolute, and may be overridden by conflicting rights claims. Thus public policy in healthcare, for example, should be guided by a cost–benefit analysis to provide a 'decent minimum' based 'on the justifiability of social expenditures rather than on some notion of natural, inalienable or pre-existing rights',[9] so that such a right would not necessarily impose an obligation on the host community.

Bell distinguishes between the negative right to health, which only implies a right not to have the present state of health (good or bad) compromised, does not carry a right to healthcare, and has no implications for treatment, and the positive right to good health which does carry such a right.[10] However, Tristram Engelhardt questions what is meant by the care necessary to achieve good health, given that for some the restoration of good health, however much care is given, is impossible, and for whom the right to good health is meaningless.[11] Daniels disputes the whole distinction between right to health and right to healthcare. He points out that 'if my poor health is not the result of anyone's doing – or failing to do – something for or to me . . . then it is hard to see how any right of mine is violated'.[3] In the context of disability this argument breaks down, since this rarely results from any person's action, so Daniels would presumably claim that no right to treatment exists. However, although treatment rarely cures, it can often improve function, so I would consider that Daniels' definition is too restrictive, and denies a right for which a case can be made.

The whole thrust of medical ethics has been more concerned with the personal doctor–patient relationship than with the concept of the institutional right to healthcare.[9,12] However, McCullough points out that the right to healthcare from institutions has a long history, dating back to eighteenth- and early-nineteenth-century Europe. He quotes Gregory's *Memorial to the Managers of The Royal Infirmary* of 1800: 'whatever it is the duty of physicians and surgeons to do to their patients, it is the duty of the managers of a hospital to procure for the sick who are admitted in it. Whatever it is the duty of physicians and surgeons not to do to their patients, it is the duty of the managers not to permit in their hospital.'[12] He nevertheless stresses the central role of the practitioner–patient relationship in that 'moral rules constitutive of medicine as a social enterprise may originate from the moral constraints on the practitioner–patient relationship as well as from social justice . . . to dismiss this . . . will be no improvement if the result is a theory for just healthcare that unjustly sacrifices individual rights for the common good'.[12]

Rights are often said to be based on autonomy, but in Judaism, for instance, autonomy is not paramount. For example, Jakobovits[13] cites a biblical source (2 Kings, Chapter 8, verses 9 and 10) to justify lying to a patient if the physician feels that to tell the truth would be harmful. If rights are vested in autonomous persons, in order that the corresponding duties can be demanded of that person and of others, it cannot be that they are exclusively so vested, since this would imply that those incapable of autonomy have no rights, excluding two subgroups of the population, namely children who are too young to exert autonomy, and those who are so disabled as to be incapable of doing so. One way round this would be to vest their autonomy in a proxy, such as the host community, who would then exercise the right on their behalf and undertake the duties. Moral rights are less precise than legal rights, which can be defined, as can the holder of the right and the person with the duty to fulfil its terms, and they often involve striking a balance between conflicting rights and duties.

Vlastos suggests that there is a right to just distribution, and that this can be considered under five headings – to each according to his need, his worth, his merit, his work and the agreement that he has made.

In an essay on *King Lear*, Ignatieff distinguishes between need and due.[14] He regards needs as common to all humans, regardless of rank (basically these needs are food, shelter and clothing). All people have an equal need for and right to these. In *King Lear*, being prepared only to provide these for their father, Goneril and Regan demean him by depriving him of that which is due to him alone as their king and father. Ignatieff argues that by only meeting basic and common needs, the dignity of the person as an individual is offended, in that he is merely an anonymous member of the human species, rather than a person with unique attributes and status which merit an unequal share. On the other hand, he points out that in the love auction, in demanding of Cordelia a profession of her love for him, Lear demands as his due that which cannot be given, namely the love of another. The question arises as to whether the unique status of, say, the Hasidic Jews makes it necessary to provide for their religious education as part of their due, which is necessary for their continued dignity, or whether in demanding it they are demanding that which cannot or should not be given.

To take a different example, namely the right of patients or their surrogates to determine treatment, then in law at least the position is not unclear. In the USA, for example, the wishes of the family of a woman in a permanent vegetative state, who wanted the continuation of treatment that the medical staff considered was futile, were upheld.[15] In the UK in some similar cases the wishes of the family were not upheld,[16] and in others, specifically the provision of special education within Hasidic schools, they were.[17]

Whether a particular treatment is appropriate for a particular patient at a particular time, or whether there are moral or ethical grounds for applying or withholding it, depends to some extent on whether the treatment is thought to be futile and, if so, whether such treatment should be colluded with. Kopelman suggests that there are four necessary conditions which must be taken into account before deciding whether a treatment is futile or of marginal benefit. First, is the treatment 'grounded in medical science'? Secondly, is the decision based on 'value-laden judgements incorporating estimates about something's utility relative to some goal, or whether the achievable goal is worth the effort'? Thirdly, is the proposed treatment 'near the threshold of . . . what is considered useless or beneficial'? Fourthly, would the treatment be 'physically, psychologically or economically burdensome'?[18] Kopelman points out that even decisions which are based on medical science are not always unanimous, and that the other three conditions are always a matter of opinion. She comes to no clear conclusion as to who should have ultimate responsibility for making the decision. The idea that the physician is the only one with the expertise necessary to decide on the value of a given therapy smacks of paternalism, but on the other hand the problem is not resolved by giving the decision to the patient or their surrogate, or to social consensus.

Gatter and Moskop discuss futility in the paradigm cases, namely the continuance of life-support treatment in patients who are in a permanent vegetative state, and intensive care for terminally ill patients.[19] They suggest that, rather than relying on a decision as to what is futile treatment, it would be better to employ a triage system, so that treatment that may not be futile, but which may be wasteful, is eliminated by public consensus. However, it would not resolve the dilemma posed by providing special support for minority groups, since this would require considerable altruism on the part of the majority for the consensus to be in their favour.

Although in the paradigms the criteria for taking one decision or the other are not always clear, the effect is. To continue life support ensures that vital functions continue, whereas to discontinue life support ensures that they do not. However, treatment of disability is only aimed at improving the patient's impaired ability to function in society. If the treatment has to be given in an unorthodox way in order to meet the specific needs of the minority group, its effectiveness may be lessened. On the other hand, if the patient is alienated from their community in order to receive adequate therapy, this must also reduce the overall effectiveness of their functioning as a member of that community. The concept of futile treatment does not advance the argument, and is fraught with difficulty because the word is used differently by different people. What one regards as futile depends to a large extent on the position that one takes vis-à-vis quality of life. Thus if an individual is best served by being fully integrated into their community, then treatment that adversely affects this is futile. On the other hand, if optimum improvement of impaired function is the main criterion, then providing sub-optimal treatment in order to accommodate cultural needs is futile.

In attempting to meet the needs of its constituents with limited and inadequate resources, a community will need to define a hierarchy of needs if the interests of the whole community are to be met, and it could be said that the availability of resources should be a criterion for deciding on the provision of treatment, and that the host is under no other obligation. At the top of the hierarchy must, of course, be the intrinsic life-sustaining universal course-of-life needs, and below it those needs which if not met will harm the community as a whole, or alternatively which if met will maximise its well-being. In order that needs can be met, the resources must be available to meet them, and the person controlling those resources must accept the obligation to meet those particular needs, but even this can cause problems in defining the community responsible. For example, in the widespread current famines the need for food is universally accepted as a course-of-life need, but hundreds of thousands are still dying because no individual community will accept the obligation to provide it.

What then is the obligation of a community (for example, the health and education services of an inner-city borough) to provide for the needs of its constituents, given that the resources are limited? To maximise the well-being of its constituents, its priority will be to provide for needs which are universal and essential (for example, food), and then to provide for those which have been accepted as necessary, as a result of legislation or general consent (for example, the provision of appropriate management and education for all children in the borough, whether they are disabled or not). Providing for special selective needs may prejudice this. If the well-being of the community as a whole is to be enhanced, then the primary factor determining which needs are to be met must be the resources available, since they inevitably determine what can be provided. Within these resources, universal course-of-life needs must be met first, since these will presumably provide for the generality of the community. Only once this has been achieved can selective aspects of needs be met.

Perceived needs are therefore not necessarily a good rule of thumb on which to distribute resources, but they are useful for judging the effectiveness of the use of resources. The extent of unmet need also provides one means of assessing the adequacy of the resources available.

Vlastos,[1] distinguishes between worth and merit. A human being has worth purely because he or she is a human being. For example, if a treatment is needed by two people and is only available to one of them, if the right to it is to be decided on the basis of worth, then they each have an equal right to it. The fact that one is young and the other old, one is rich and the other poor, one is clever and the other foolish, or even that one is an upright citizen of great benefit to the community and the other a vicious criminal, cannot be taken into account. They are both human beings, and therefore of equal worth. However, no two people will be of equal merit, since this depends not on their humanity, nor even on their abilities, but on what they have achieved with the cards that have been dealt them. A father may count his two sons equally worthy of his love, but may feel that the one who has worked hard is of greater merit than the one who has wasted his substance. Nevertheless, the fatted calf was killed for the prodigal son on the basis of his worth as a human being and son of the house, rather than on his merit as a diligent and hard-working farmer (Luke, Chapter 15, verses 11–32). This relates to Ignatieff's concept of due rather than need. Lear was due additional care from his daughters because he was their father and king, irrespective of whether his performance in those roles was good, bad or indifferent.

The idea of rights being allocated according to works performed is related to the above. However, the contribution that my work makes to the community must reflect not only my merit – what use I make of the skills that I have – but also the quality of those skills. If my skills are intrinsically poor, however meritoriously I employ them they will contribute little to the general good, and therefore few rights will accrue from them.

Vlastos' final category, namely the right to be provided for according to the agreement one has made, relates directly to the fulfilment of obligations. In considering the interests of the child, it is necessary to take a holistic approach. The child exists in a family, within a culture and within a community, and any agreements that are made on his or her behalf will involve all three of these groupings. It is fashionable to describe the UK as a multicultural society. This is related to what Ignatieff[20] describes as civic nationalism. All people within a geographical area, regardless of their inheritance, culture or ethnicity, subscribe to the nation state, and are bound by its laws and customs. He contrasts this with what he calls ethnic nationalism, in which the group is defined precisely by ethnicity and inherited culture, independent of geography.

There are many groups within the UK whose primary loyalty is to a cultural group that is separate from the nation state, and often extends outside its borders. It is thus not so much a multicultural society as a society of multiple cultures. For example, second- and third-generation Bangladeshi children are regularly taken back to Bangladesh for a period of months in order to retain their hold on their family culture and language, even if this means that the visit coincides with examinations that they have worked for, or even if they take the examinations, but the lost schooling involved means that they are twice as likely to fail them as their compatriots who do not take such unauthorised leave.[21] Failure to maintain their identity as Bangladeshis is seen as a greater loss than failure to gain the means of advancing in our society.

The Hasids are another such community. The primary authority is the Law of God as revealed in the scriptures, but the primary earthly authority is the Rebbe of that particular sect. These two authorities, divine and human, result in the closed communities in which the Hasids live. This exclusiveness is not new. Singer begins his novel, *Shosha*, the story of a Hasid boy in pre-Nazi Warsaw, as follows: 'I was brought up on three dead languages . . . and in a culture that developed in Babylon: the Talmud. The cheder where I studied was a room in which the teacher ate and slept, and his wife cooked. There I studied not arithmetic . . . but the laws governing an egg laid on a holiday . . . Although my ancestors had settled in Poland some six or seven hundred years before I was born, I knew only a few words of the Polish language'.[22] Even more than the Bangladeshis, this community transcends national boundaries, and it is not uncommon for families to move within the community to different nation states. If one is to consider the disabled Hasidic child holistically, then their need to be part of the cultural group is important. However, they do live in the secular state of the UK, and they benefit from its infrastructure. In gaining the legal right to the benefits provided by the state, they also gain a legal duty to abide by the laws and rules of conduct in that country.

Therefore when deciding what rights accrue to individuals within a group such as the Hasidim, it is necessary to consider all five of Vlastos' categories, not only their needs. Their worth as human beings will afford them the same rights as any other member of the community. It may be that they have an additional right that is their due, in Ignatieff's sense – to maintain their dignity not just as human beings, but as human beings in a particular role, namely that of Hasids. As far as merit (the contribution that they and their group have made to the community which is providing for the right) is concerned, this is more difficult, since as a group they tend to be inward-looking and make little overt contribution to the general community. On the other hand, they cause little disruption, tend to be law abiding in the secular as well as the religious sense, and take little from the general community.

The latter point does relate to what form the contract or agreement that they have with the wider community, as part of that wider community, should take. As well as being members of their own communities, they are also members of the wider community, and have duties as well as rights within that community.

In summary, therefore, it is in the interests of the host community that needs are met so far as is possible. The first priority must be given to universal course-of-life needs. Secondly, those needs that have been accepted as equivalent to universal course-of-life needs by statute or mutual agreement must be met. As far as resources allow, attempts should also be made to meet specific, non-universal course-of-life needs. In this way the well-being of the whole community can be safeguarded by maximising the well-being of individuals within that community.

References

1 Vlastos G (1984) Justice and equality. In: J Waldron (ed.) *Theories of Rights.* Oxford University Press, Oxford, pp. 41–76.

2 Childress JF (1979) A right to health care? *J Med Phil.* **4**: 132–47.

3 Daniels N (1979) Rights to health care and distributive justice: programmatic worries. *J Med Phil.* **4**: 174–91.

4 Beauchamp TL and Childress JE (1983) *Principles of Biomedical Ethics* (2e). Oxford University Press, New York.

5 Wiggins D and Derman S (1987) Needs, need, needing. *J Med Ethics.* **13**: 62–8.

6 Lockwood M (1981) Words: rights. *J Med Ethics.* **7**: 150–2.

7 Waldron J (1984) Introduction. In: J Waldron (ed.) *Theories of Rights.* Oxford University Press, Oxford, pp. 1–20.

8 Shelton RL (1978) Human rights and distributive justice in health care issues. *J Med Ethics.* **4**: 165–71.

9 Beauchamp TL and Faden RR (1979) The right to health and the right to health care. *J Med Phil.* **4**: 118–31.

10 Bell NK (1979) The scarcity of medical resources: are there rights to health care? *J Med Phil.* **4**: 158–69.

11 Tristram Engelhardt H (1979) Rights to health care: a critical appraisal. *J Med Phil.* **4**: 113–17.

12 McCullough LB (1979) Rights, health care and public policy. *J Med Phil.* **4**: 204–15.

13 Jakobovits I (1986) The Jewish contribution to medical ethics. In: P Byrne (ed.) *Rights and Wrongs in Medicine.* King's Fund, London, pp. 115–26.

14 Ignatieff M (1984) *The Needs of Strangers.* Chatto and Windus Ltd, London.

15 Cranford RE, Rie ME and Ackerman F (1991) Helga Wanglie's ventilator. *Hastings Cent Rep.* **21**: 23–9.

16 Dyer C (1987) Going to law to get treatment. *BMJ.* **295**: 1554.

17 Regina v The Inner London Education Authority ex parte F. (Unreported case. Transcript reference CO\365\88.)

18 Kopelman LM (1995) Conceptual and moral disputes about futile and useful treatments. *J Med Phil.* **20**: 109–21.

19 Gatter RA and Moskop JC (1995) From futility to triage. *J Med Phil.* **20**: 191–205.

20 Ignatieff M (1994) *Blood and Belonging.* Vintage, London.

21 Gloun N (1998) Long visits abroad could cost pupils places. *Times Educ Suppl.* **4255**: 19.

22 Singer IB (1995) Shosha. In: *Three Complete Novels.* Wings Books, Avenel, NJ, pp. 295–454.

Chapter 11

Conclusions

An attempt has been made to define the ethical considerations inherent in working with a group within society which does not share the generally held beliefs of that society, and which judges priorities on a different system of values. The specific problem considered has been that posed by attempting simultaneously to meet what are seen as the medical and educational needs of disabled children within the group, and to accommodate the group's beliefs.

Although it is usually, but not always, possible to define impairment in precise anatomical or physiological terms, disability and handicap are much more subjective, and dependent on the perceptions of the person involved and the society in which he or she lives. In a wider context, the perceptions that society has of a disabled person are as much influenced by fears and prejudices as by the actual restrictions that the impairment places on that person. I have commented on legally enshrined restrictions placed on disabled people in Germany, but this is by no means confined to that country. Silvers comments that much testimony supporting the passage of the 1990 Americans with Disabilities Act related to various legal decisions in the USA that, for example, 'barred, maimed, mutilated or otherwise deformed individuals from . . . public places' or excluded a boy with cerebral palsy from school because 'he produced a depressing and nauseating effect on the teachers and school children'.[1] Recent legislation in most western countries, like the above Act, has helped people with disabilities to combat such prejudice, but nevertheless what constitutes a disability and the handicap which it entails is very much embedded in the cultural responses to it not only of the community at large, but also the disabled person him- or herself.

What perhaps causes disability and handicap to a greater extent than anything else is being the outsider – being the one who cannot manage in society as it happens to be constituted. In *The Country of the Blind*,[2] by HG Wells, it is not the fact that the mountaineer has eyes which disables him. It is the fact that his other senses are insufficiently developed to enable him to function in the same way that the other people of the valley function – he is literally the outsider. The apparent physical deformity for that society, the impairment for them – the eyes – is the feature about him that can be used to explain his disability, and which can thereby provide an apparent means of curing him of it. Removing his eyes would give him a semblance of what in that community is physical normality, even though it would cause him even greater disability by removing the one sense – sight – which enables him to cope at all. Treating him in this way – rendering him normal by the standards of that community – removes the need for the other members of the community to alter their own way of life in order to adjust to his problems. This is at the heart of Oliver's comments about the able-bodied in society believing that the disabled should aspire to normality however that happens to be defined by the host community,[3] and my comments on facial plastic surgery in babies with Down syndrome, that it is performed to attempt to normalise the child's facial appearance.[4] How the community is constituted, and what is considered to be a failure to function normally, are largely defined by the secular and religious culture of that community, which raises the question of whether insisting, for example, that a Hasidic child be treated in a secular school causes him to be an outsider in his own community, and this therefore becomes more of a handicap than his cerebral palsy or Down syndrome.

Although what are claimed to be the teachings of the religion of the community are often used to define attitudes to disability, other factors play a large role. Intimately linked to religious attitudes is what often amounts to superstition that is loosely based on the religion, which sees the problem in terms of divine or demonic visitation, or the response to some personal or communal failure. Many of the miracles of Jesus are portrayed in terms of casting out devils that were causing epilepsy or unsocial behaviour (for example, the casting out of devils into the Gadarene swine; Matthew, Chapter 8, verses 28–32).[5] Furthermore, if there is a real or perceived penalty for the family in having a disabled member, such as ostracism from the community or restriction on marriage of other members of the family, this will greatly influence the perception of disabled people and their management by the family.

In this context, much of the causation of disability is seen in terms of guilt. This may be universal, resulting perhaps from the fall of Adam, familial, providing a justified punishment for the sins of the parents, or personal, for example, in the doctrine of karma, with present disability resulting from sins committed and unresolved in past incarnations. If it is believed to be the result of guilt, then disability is a cause for shame and punishment, so that this again influences attitudes to the disabled person and his or her family, and justifies ostracism.

Anything that influences the perception of disability will inevitably influence the way in which treatment is accepted. If the disabled person is to be treated effectively, then the treatment has to be accepted by that person or his or her carers. Whether the treatment consists of advice or medication, if it is not taken it is wasted. The treatment is more likely to be acceptable if it is holistic – if it treats the person as a whole, rather than as the sum of their parts, or even worse, as only part of the sum of their parts. The whole will involve not only the person, but also that person in his environment and community, and this will include consideration of his own beliefs about the causation and meaning of his disability. This exacerbates the problem, since a physician who ignores this aspect of treatment by taking no note of the patient's beliefs will compromise his or her treatment. On the other hand, although it is almost a cliché to assume that the beliefs of others must be respected at all times, no belief system can be given carte blanche so that, whatever the outcome, the patient's beliefs must be the overriding factor determining treatment. There are clearly circumstances in which the beliefs may be so abhorrent, or the effect of following them so damaging to others as well as to the patient himself, that this policy cannot be adopted.

It is necessary to examine the circumstances under which beliefs should be respected and thus taken into account when planning patient management. If they either pose too great a burden on the wider community, or result in such disruption of the treatment that they harm the child, then it may be necessary to insist that they be violated. This need not put an insuperable barrier between the secular and the religious since, in Judaism in particular, this can to some extent be justified in that the overriding criterion is to save life, and even the law of God can be broken in order to achieve this. However, this involves the extreme case of saving a life. Lesser problems, such as the management of disability, are unlikely to be resolved by such agreement between the religious and secular authorities. In the case of disabled children, such resolution requires consideration not only of the benefit or harm that adherence to the belief may bring to the individual and to the wider society, but also of the question of who has the authority to decide, since the subjects are usually incompetent to do so themselves. This is not to say that disputes are bound to arise in all cases. The question of who has the authority to decide is only of importance if there is disagreement between the parties. If the criteria for respecting the beliefs can be met, and this does not result in actual harm to the child or impose an unreasonable burden on the wider community, no problem need arise. However, the definition of harm, and what in a particular situation constitutes harm, is not easy to decide, and there is a need to evaluate the relative effect of different harms in order to achieve a balance of harm. This is particularly pertinent to evaluating the relative weight to be placed on the harm caused by receiving suboptimal treatment, as opposed to the harm due to being excluded from full membership of one's family and religious community.

The contract between the doctor and the patient is not one-sided – the doctor has rights as well as the patient. Thus the effect that adherence to a particular belief may have on the actual treatment that can be offered, in particular whether the effect is so great and the treatment so compromised that the physician cannot collude with it without compromising his own integrity, or his duty to others in the wider community, also has to be considered. Again there is often a need to achieve a balance of harms, so that it may be appropriate to opt for adequate although less effective treatment in the short term, in order to prevent, for example, the long-term harm of being excluded from the family. The key here is that the treatment, although less effective, is nevertheless effective, and can be applied ethically. For example, a case can be made to attempt to induce a remission in leukaemia without using blood transfusion, even though this has a lower likelihood of success than other methods, in order to prevent the long-term rejection of the child by their Jehovah's Witness parents.[5] However, it would be considerably more difficult to accede to a request to circumcise or infibulate a young girl in order to ensure that she would be accepted as a marriage partner by the men of her community in adulthood, since these operations have no therapeutic value, and for most people outside the girl's community they constitute an unreasonable assault and mutilation.

If acting on a belief causes harm to the person who holds that belief, to others in the community or to the community at large, and this harm is not outweighed by any coincident social advantage, it is difficult to respect that belief. Since it is not always possible to avoid all harms, a balance must be struck in order to avoid greater harm even if a lesser harm ensues. In deciding who speaks for the child, weight must be given to the child's opinions, even if technically they are not competent, as well as to those of the parents. Only if there is disagreement between the health or educational authorities and these two agents, and if a greater harm would ensue by adhering to the wishes of the latter than by overriding them, do problems of consent arise. Although a physician or other therapist is under no obligation to compromise his or her own integrity and rights by colluding with bad, ineffective or dangerous treatment, he or she should make every effort to accommodate the wishes and beliefs of the patient and their family.

In any form of treatment, particularly that involved in the treatment of disability, the contract between the treated and the treater is not the only contract involved. There are also wider contracts, not only between the disabled person and the host community that is providing the resources needed for treatment but, in the type of situation under discussion here, between the minority community and the host community. Each party has both rights and responsibilities under the contract. Clearly the host community has the same obligations to the minority culture that it has to any other group or individual within its jurisdiction, and it is required, for example, to comply with the law both as it applies to the provision of resources generally, and as may be decided in particular cases.[6] This may involve providing resources in such a way that the overall availability is diminished, for example, if staff have to be diverted to provide services within the group's schools. However, it is questionable whether there is always an obligation to provide services over and above those provided to the general population in order to accommodate the specific needs of the group – needs that the general population does not have. This distinction between specific rights and general rights may be spurious, since if the one can be converted to the other by rewording the question that is asked, the difference between the two is diminished. However, it could be argued that acknowledging the need to reword the question gives tacit support to the fact that there is a problem for the minority group that is not a problem for the host group.

However, the contract is reciprocal and the minority community has obligations towards the host community. Whether or not they claim rights which may involve them receiving a disproportionate amount of resources, they do form a constituent part of the host community and have an obligation to conform to the requirements of that community unless they can produce convincing evidence that this would cause them harm. It cannot be claimed that there is always a duty to comply with the law. Clearly, for example, Jews were under no obligation to conform to the anti-Semitic laws of Nazi Germany. Furthermore, the Nuremberg Tribunals established that the claim that one was obeying the law in force at the time, or obeying orders, was not a defence if the result was the sort of crimes against humanity that were perpetrated by the Third Reich. Bad laws must not only not be obeyed – they must also be actively resisted. The problem is knowing by what criteria one can decide that a law is bad. In retrospect, laws which ban Jews from holding public office and which pave the way to the massacre of an entire people cannot be seen as anything but infamous. However, if skilfully presented, would they have appeared so in prospect, given that the 'Final Solution of the Jewish Problem' would not initially be seen as following from them? I still vividly remember a lesson taught by a supply teacher 50 years ago. He asked us to comment on a newspaper article on separate development in South Africa, a new system that was being introduced, in which the various nations which made up the country would have their own areas in which they could pursue their own culture – a system called apartheid, a word that was then quite new to us. To the consternation of the teacher, none of the intelligent 13-year-olds in the class could see anything wrong with it, although now most would regard it as a great evil comparable to Nazism. This was a time when the West Indian immigration to this country had only just begun, and cinema newsreels on how they were settling in commonly showed them turning up at Anglican churches and being kindly directed to their own churches, where they would be 'more comfortable'. Even more nakedly racist were advertisements for rooms to let, which commonly contained the phrase 'No blacks'. It was also a time when it was considered quite acceptable, despite the Holocaust, for golf clubs, etc., to advertise openly that Jewish members were not allowed. In such a climate apartheid seemed benign.

Deciding in extreme situations is relatively easy, but it is less easy to know to what extent one is entitled to disobey (either in letter or in spirit) less extreme laws with which one disagrees, or which offend some aspect of one's culture. For example, two laws which require the wearing of a crash helmet when riding a motorbike and a hard hat when on construction sites offend Sikhs.[7,8] Both of these measures significantly reduce the risk of the individual sustaining a severe head injury should an accident occur. On one level it might be said that whether or not one chooses to protect oneself against injury is a personal matter that does not require the intervention of the State, and indeed such intervention is an unwarranted interference with personal freedom and should be resisted. However, there is a public interest to be considered. The cost to the community in time, money and resources of long-term care for people disabled by severe head injury is enormous, and it could be argued that the community, through its laws, has the right to protect itself against such cost, and that individuals within the State accept the duty of protecting the community by protecting themselves. In this case, the problem is resolved by allowing Sikhs to wear the turban in place of a crash helmet or hard hat,[8,9] but with the clear statement in the Employment Act that if injury occurs, compensation will be on the basis of an estimate of the injury that would have occurred had a crash helmet or hard hat been worn. In other words, the law has been modified to take account of the cultural needs of the Sikhs, but imposes on them a duty to avoid increasing the burden on other parties, although this is only partial in that it is tacitly assumed that the injury they would receive is likely to be more severe than it would be if they were wearing a hard hat.

It is in this area – the restriction of personal freedom for the good of the community – that the potential for bad law exists. In a democracy, laws are enacted by the elected Government, which in turn reflects the views of that section of the community (not necessarily the majority) that elected it, rather than the views of the whole community. The rights of minorities, particularly unpopular minorities, are likely to be over-looked. For example, the above Acts take account of the needs of the Sikhs, a vocal, well-respected minority, but not those of the Rastafarians, a less vocal, less respected group whose objection to the prescribed headgear is identical to that of the Sikhs – it offends their religion.

However, laws such as those governing, for example, the health and safety of children in a school, or the quality of the education that is provided, apply to and are to the benefit of all children of the majority and minority communities alike. The minority group, if asking for resources from the majority community, should be required to conform to these laws. This is not easy to apply in practice. For example, many of the buildings that the Hasidic community use as their schools are admitted by them to be inadequate (schmaterlich in the words of the *Times Educational Supplement*).[10] To bring them up to the necessary standard would be extremely costly and probably beyond the resources of the communities involved. If the majority community is going to demand this, it could be that there is an obligation on them to help with the cost, again of course at potential detriment to the resources available to the rest of the community. Once more there is by no means clear agreement as to what constitutes acceptable standards of educa-tion, and to insist, for example, that the standards of a national curric-ulum must be met could actually impinge on the religious needs of the group. Although these could seem to be insurmountable obstacles, as has been demonstrated in the compromises that have been made over headgear for Sikhs,[9] a compromise could probably be reached.

In attempting to reach such a compromise, the interests and rights of five agencies need to be considered, namely the child patient, the parent, the physician, the minority community and the host community. This can be made easier if it can be established within these five agencies which interests have priority. There seems to be general agreement that the welfare of the patient is paramount, even though there may not be agreement as to how this can best be safeguarded. For example, even when discussing the doctor in a non-medical role, in health service management, the claim is that this 'starts from the premise that the principal concern of everyone involved in the delivery of health services must be the care, treatment and safety of patients'.[11] Therefore in any such prioritisation the interests and rights of the patient must be at its head.

In the same publication, it is stated that 'Public health physicians must make the health of their population their main concern'.[11] The clear implication here is that all physicians have a responsibility to look to all of their patients. Indeed, the first quotation refers to 'patients', not 'the patient'. I therefore put the interests of the host community second.

If an accommodation can be made which meets the interests and rights of these two agencies, this will meet most of the rights of the parent and the physician. If with adjustment the latter rights can be fully met, then these will in turn meet most of the interests and rights of the minority community.

The interests and rights of the patient fall into two broad categories – medical and general. The medical interests are fairly straightforward. The treatment that is proposed must be appropriate, and any harm that may result from it can only be justified if it is outweighed by the benefits. The patient must be given sufficient information to enable him or her to understand the treatment and its implications, and in the case of a young child, they must have the support of an appropriate adult carer, usually the parent. Given that there is in fact a disorder in need of treatment, and that the child will derive benefit from the treatment, I would suggest that the above needs fit the criteria for course-of-life needs. Failure to meet them would therefore constitute a course-of-life harm.

The general interests are also important. If a child is to thrive, she needs to be nurtured within a stable family, within a stable culture and within the host community. Failure to meet these needs would also constitute course-of-life harm. Implicit in this is a need to attend schools that are acceptable to the particular group to which the family belongs. However, there is no cultural requirement that the schools should be inadequate, for example, that they should not comply with legal health and safety requirements, or that the teachers should not be competent in the basic skills of pedagogy. Since secular studies are usually allowed, there is also no reason why they should not be required to fulfil the requirements of the National Curriculum.

As far as the interests of the host community are concerned, these will be met if the interests of the individuals and groups within the community are maximised with the resources available. This involves preventing course-of-life harm by meeting, so far as is possible, at least the course-of-life needs of the community. A distinction has been made between universal course-of-life needs and group-specific course-of-life needs, and there is a tacit assumption that the former take precedence over the latter. However, can such a distinction be sustained? It could be claimed that failure to meet specific course-of-life needs causes such harm that it affects the whole community. Certainly failure to meet the primary course-of-life need, the continuance of life itself, for the specific communities of Jews and Gypsies in the Third Reich has had a profound and continuing effect on the whole world community to this day. Could failure to meet lesser course-of-life needs, for example, for group-specific education in order to respect religious conviction, be equally damaging to the host community? It has the potential to seem discriminatory, and it is certainly viewed as such by the community.[10]

How then can the needs of the child and of the host community be simultaneously met? The problem is not that the child needs treatment which differs from that of the other children in the community. The problem is that the requirements of the religious belief, for example, separate treatment groups for male and female children, male therapists at boys' schools, etc., mean that the treatment is much more costly in terms of time, money and resources. It has been argued that the unequal distribution of available resources is justified in order to prevent a course-of-life harm. Examples would include the protection afforded Salman Rushdie against the fatwah, or that afforded to political leaders. If it is accepted that taking notice of the religious beliefs of the child and his or her family is in the child's interest and, as discussed above, also impinges on the wider host community interest, then there is an obligation on the wider community to meet this need.

On the other hand, the interests of the individual within the host community are dependent on the interests of the whole community. Part of this wider interest is that the laws of the host community which are not unjust should be obeyed. Arising from this, I would argue that the minority community has an obligation to ensure that its specific agencies (schools, etc.) do adhere to these laws as discussed above.

The interests of the physician are served if they can fulfil their obligations to provide effective and ethical treatment for their patients, and are not required to collude with ineffective, unethical treatment. If a compromise can be reached as described above, whereby the child receives adequate treatment from the host community, and the religious community adheres to the laws regarding, for example, health and safety, then the child should receive adequate therapy. If such a compromise can be reached, the interests of the physician will be automatically safeguarded.

Similarly, the interests of the parents will also be safeguarded. Their religious beliefs will be respected, their child will receive appropriate treatment, and they will be able to participate in decisions that are made about their child without compromising their adherence to a minority culture.

Since the child and their family would, as a result of this solution, receive treatment comparable to that received by any other member of the host community, without requiring them to compromise their membership of a minority religious group, the interests of the group would also be protected.

What then of the specific question of there being a duty on the medical and educational services of the host community to comply with the demands for resources to be used to benefit disabled children in minority communities, by accepting the need to respect the religious needs of the communities as well as the medical and educational needs of the child, even though this may result in an overall reduction in the availability of resources for all children? I have argued that there is such a duty, provided that the minority community complies with the reasonable demands of the host community, as discussed above. If the minority community is not prepared to meet the above demands, so that complying with their religious needs potentially results in condoning poor or even dangerous levels of treatment and education, then in my view it is unreasonable for the resources of the host community to be so diverted.

References

1 Silvers A (1996) (In)equality, (ab)normality, and the Americans with Disabilities Act. *J Med Phil.* **21**: 209–24.

2 Wells HG (1967) The country of the blind. Reprinted in: C Dolley (ed.) *The Penguin Book of English Short Stories.* Penguin, Harmondsworth, pp. 103–28.

3 Oliver M (1989) Conductive education: if it wasn't so sad it would be funny. *Disabil Handicap Soc.* **4**: 197–200.

4 Jones RB (2000) Point of view: parental consent to cosmetic facial surgery in Down's Syndrome. *J Med Ethics.* **26**:101–2.

5 Kearney PJ (1978) Leukaemia in children of Jehovah's Witnesses: issues and priorities in a conflict of care. *J Med Ethics.* **4**: 32–5.

6 Regina v Inner London Education Authority ex parte F. (Unreported case. Transcript reference CO\365\88.)

7 *Road Traffic Act 1972.* C20. Section 32. HMSO, London.

8 *Employment Act 1989.* C38. Section 11. HMSO, London.

9 *Motor-Cycle Crash Helmets (Religious Exemptions) Act 1976.* C62. HMSO, London.

10 Wallace W (1988) Why is our school so schmaterlich, Daddy? *Times Educ Suppl.* **5 February**.

11 General Medical Council (1999) *Management in Health Care: the Role of Doctors.* General Medical Council, London, p. 5.

Index